AF344462

RADIOLOGY OF
FACIAL INJURY

RADIOLOGY OF FACIAL INJURY

Second Edition

Kenneth D. Dolan, M.D.
Charles G. Jacoby, M.D.
Wendy R. K. Smoker, M.D.

Department of Radiology
University Hospitals and Clinics
Iowa City, Iowa

Macmillan Publishing Company
New York

Collier Macmillan Canada, Inc.
Toronto

Collier Macmillan Publishers
London

Distributed by:
Macmillan Publishing Company
866 Third Avenue, New York, NY 10022

Collier Macmillan Canada, Inc.
Collier Macmillan Publishers • London

Library of Congress Catalog Card Number: 87-082577
ISBN 0-02-329941-X

Printing: 1   2   3   4   5   6   7
Year: 7   8   9   0   1   2   3

Preface

This book represents a summation of a large experience with the study of facial injury spanning more than twenty years of consultation about the radiologic aspects of these injuries. Our hospital complex serves as the tertiary center for the care of some 2.5 million people. Not only do we have a pool of simple injuries from our local college town inhabitants but also we have a broad referral area from which many intermediate, complex, and multiple injuries are referred for care.

The radiologist fits into the facial injury care role somewhat like the conductor of an orchestra composed of those who perform definitive care of these patients. Frequently the emergency room physician is the first to see the facial injury patient. With the information gained from primary radiological evaluation, the emergency physician can then add the services of the otolaryngologist, oral surgeon, ophthalmologist and oculoplastic surgeon, maxillofacial, and plastic surgeon as needed. Accompanying medical problems bring the aspects of facial injury further into the province of the neurologist, neurosurgeon, anesthesiologist, orthopedist, and intensive care physician.

It is up to the radiologist then to devise and interpret the various examinations which enable the treatment group to collect pertinent basic information needed to evaluate their concerns about the injured patient.

This book serves as a means of directing the radiologic inquiry and provides the anatomic and pathologic background necessary to evaluate facial injuries.

Our study began in 1965 when the senior author was asked to present a radiological correlation in a maxillofacial injury course given by a former otolaryngologic colleague, Dr. Leslie Bernstein. Since the course was to include laboratory demonstrations of surgical facial injury care, we undertook an attempt to create common injuries in anatomic materials available to us. Nasal and zygomatic arch injuries were easy to produce. However, even by following the directions described in the LeFort papers, it was nearly impossible to specifically create the injuries he described. This impressed us in respect to the strength and resiliency of the facial skeleton and stimulated Kenneth Dolan to study facial radiologic anatomy critically and develop criteria of facial injury from radiographic studies.

Multidirectional tomography was being developed by this time and became a helpful tool to uncover hidden or only slightly displaced fractures and gave, at least, a suggestion of soft tissue changes accompanying the skeletal alterations.

Charles Jacoby joined our faculty and developed an interest in head and neck radiology about the time that computerized tomography (CT) became available. From the crude beginnings of 64 × 64 matrix first generation equipment, our interest and enthusiasm grew in proportion to the increasing resolution afforded by improved CT equipment. Bone displacement revealed by axial CT examination with coronal and sagittal reformatting gave us a new dimension of fragment analysis which was further applied to our conventional and tomographic radiographic analysis. CT also provided a large contribution to the evaluation of the orbit and ocular structures in injury.

By this time our ideas had been presented to a number of maxillofacial injury conferences and radiological departments throughout the country. Dolan and Jacoby were asked to prepare a summary article on maxillofacial injury for *Seminars in Radiology* by Dr. Ben Felson. This material was incorporated with other articles, in a second issue, to form an overview of the principles of radiologic evaluation of fractures in book form. This article allowed us to at least outline our ideas but did not allow presentation in depth.

Wendy Smoker was added to our team during her radiology residency, neuroradiology fellowship and as a faculty member in our department. Her work has led us to greater concern about neural injury accompanying facial injury and has encouraged us to more aggressively image and study brain and cranial nerve damage accompanying facial injury.

During this time Dolan was asked to give a two-hour refresher course on facial injury to radiologists attending the annual Radiologic Society of North America meeting. The course provided an impetus to present some of our ideas in detail. Also, each year new questions were asked by participants so that stimulus for further study and revision of our material was provided. Several times the RSNA tried to produce a slide-tape presentation of this material for postgraduate study but, for various reasons, the material could not be adopted to this format.

Finally, Dr. William Tuddenham, editor of *RadioGraphics*, an RSNA publication, assembled our material into a pictorial monograph which was published as the July 1984 volume of his journal.

This second edition of "Radiology of Facial Injuries" has a more complete accompanying text. Many additions, particularly in the area of CT correlative views and concepts, have been made. We have also included a new section related to our findings in connection with CT and magnetic resonance imaging of brain injury accompanying facial trauma.

We feel that the material now presents a comprehensive look at the radiological elements of facial injury and yet is arranged so that it also serves as a reference guide to the radiology of specific injury patterns which the radiologist and his colleagues may wish to assess.

Contents

1
Introduction

Facial injury constitutes a frequent finding among emergency room patients. Schultz and Oldham estimate that 54% of such patients will have significant trauma.

The complexity of facial structures and their relative vulnerability make it important for the radiologist to have an excellent understanding of facial osseous anatomy and patterns of injury.

The injury pattern produced varies with the degree of force applied and with the facial portion in contact with the blow. Variations may also occur as a result of the size of the object that strikes the face.

Facial injury evaluation plays a small role in the severely injured patients' overall evaluation. Survey tabletop frontal and lateral views may suffice to detect the presence of an injury that can be more completely studied when the patient has reached a stable condition.

We customarily use a 25 × 30 cm film size in our maxillofacial evaluation and advise against the use of small coned-down views such as those used for sinus studies. Ideally, the Waters and Caldwell views should be obtained as posteroanterior (PA) views so that the facial bones are best defined by being close to the film. The PA projection also gives the best representation of the orbital, maxillary, and zygomatic structures that diverge from back to front.

Complex motion tomography is preferable for facial injury evaluation, since blurring of overlying structures is most complete and parasite lines are minimized with this system. We use tomography to display details of injury that are obscure or suspected on plain film views. Tomography may also be of value in studying the extent of injury in patients who, because of multiple injuries, cannot cooperate for routine views.

Computerized tomography (CT) has also become significant in evaluating facial injury. Intraorbital and retrobulbar hematomas are difficult to detect by conventional means, but are easily displayed by CT. Similarly, bone detail and displacement may be clearly demonstrated by "bone mode" CT examination. Reconstruction of coronal and sagittal images by CT also may be very important, although sometimes the seriously injured patient may not be able to hold still long enough to permit reconstruction of axial image information.

Coronal computerized tomography may be helpful to evaluate structures that lie in a relatively axial plane, such as the hard palate, orbital floor, and orbital roof. As mentioned above, movement by the distressed patient or associated injury elsewhere may make reconstruction in either the coronal or sagittal projection impossible.

Direct coronal CT imaging may be possible in the patient with an uncomplicated injury such as a blowout fracture of the orbit floor. It seems to make little difference anatomically if the patient is placed in the supine position with the neck hyperextended or in the prone position. The choice of the position may depend on the type of machine used. We customarily tip the CT machine gantry to obtain as near coronal views as possible, however it is nearly impossible to obtain exact coronal slices. The problems are similar to those encountered in obtaining coronal views of the sella turcica.

The purpose of any radiographic study of the patient with facial injury is to provide the surgeon with information regarding the major interruptions of the facial skeleton and any displacement of the fracture fragment that may be present. Surgical techniques of fracture reduction and stabilization are based on such information.

Similarly, neural injury may be suggested by the location of a fracture or occassionally may be demonstrated directly by CT. Cerebrospinal fluid leaks may result from fractures of the frontal, ethmoidal, or sphenoidal sinus walls. Early in the course of injury, hematoma or soft tissue herniation may occlude the injury site. The radiologist may suggest the potential of such a leak when the central sinus walls are interrupted.

1. NORMAL SKELETAL ANATOMY

The facial skeleton arises from and is attached to the anterior cranial fossa and the sphenoidal bones. The broad frontal bones have indentations produced by the frontal lobe gyri as seen from above in Figure 1. The paired cribriform plates divide the central frontal surface. The crista galli is located between the cribriform plates. The falx cerebri arises from the crista galli and is attached along a vertical ridge lying behind the frontal sinuses.

A. Orbits

The orbital cavities are conical and have a central axis that diverges obliquely about 35° from the midline. The orbital axis projects downward about 15° from the posterior apex to the anterior rim.

The orbital roof primarily consists of the yoke-like frontal bone. Near the orbital apex the lesser sphenoidal wings complete the roof and form the upper margin of the superior orbital fissure.

Perpendicular curved surfaces form the medial and lateral orbital walls. The ethmoidal sinus complex forms the principal medial surface of the orbit. This surface is known as the *lamina papyracea*. Posteriorly, this surface

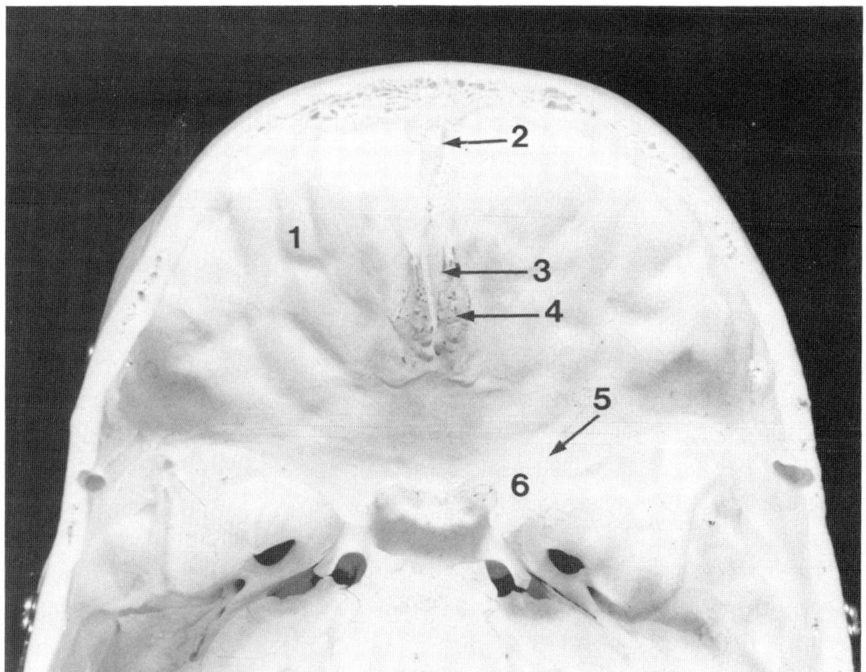

Figure 1. View of the anterior fossa from above. 1. Cerebral surface of frontal bone. 2. Falcine crest. 3. Crista galli. 4. Cribriform plate. 5. Junction of frontal bone and lesser wing. 6. Lesser wing of sphenoidal bone and anterior clinoid process.

merges with the lateral wall of the sphenoidal sinus. Anteriorly, the lamina papyracea joins the lacrimal bone. This merges with the frontal process of the maxilla, which is attached to the nasal bones.

The posterior two-thirds of the lateral orbital wall is formed by the greater sphenoidal wing and its orbital process. The orbital process of the zygoma comprises the anterior one-third of the lateral orbital wall. Both sphenoidal and zygomatic contributions are attached to the orbital process of the frontal bone.

The orbital floor, formed by the maxillary roof, is sigmoid shaped from back to front. The anterior floor is concave mediolaterally from the maxillary junction with the lamina papyracea to the maxillary process of the zygoma. Posteriorly, the inferior orbital fissure separates the maxillary and greater sphenoidal wing surfaces of the orbit. The infraorbital neurovascular structures pass through a groove in the posterior one-half of the orbital floor. Anteriorly, the infraorbital neurovascular structures pass through an enclosed canal just below the orbital floor and exit through the infraorbital foramen.

Since the orbital floor is only a thin layer of bone, it provides little skeletal support and depends on the maxillary and zygomatic thickened portions of the inferior orbital rim for support.

B. Zygomatic Arches

The curved zygomatic arches form horizontal buttresses extending from the body of the zygoma to the temporal process of the zygomatic arch. The temporal portion arises from a condensation of bone just above the glenoid fossa of the temporomandibular joint.

C. Maxillae

The anterior, nasal, and posterolateral maxillary sinus walls form a pyramidal shape in axial section. An anterior buttress forms the nasal fossa margin. Laterally, thickening extends from the zygoma to the alveolar arch. Posterior strengthening is produced by the fused pterygoid process of the sphenoid.

The convex dental alveolar portions of the maxilla are attached to the convex hard palate that forms a horizontal supporting structure.

The perpendicular bony nasal septum is formed by the ethmoidal perpendicular plate and the vomer. This provides tenuous vertical support for the nasal bones and hard palate.

2. RADIOGRAPHIC ANATOMY

A. The Caldwell (Occipitofrontal) View

The Caldwell projection should be made with the central ray directed about 25° below the canthomeatal plane to allow visualization of the orbital floor above the petrous ridge.

The following list of anatomic features is given in a suggested sequence of studying Figure 2A.

  1. Zygomaticofrontal suture
  2. Orbital process of frontal bone
  3. Anterior orbital roof
  4. Upper (palpable) orbital rim
  5. Frontal sinus
  6. Lamina papyracea
  7. Posterior orbital floor
  8. Posterior lacrimal crest
  9. Anterior orbital floor
10. Frontal process of maxilla
11. Lateral nasal wall
12. Lateral maxillary wall
13. Hard palate
14. Perpendicular ethmoid plate and vomer
15. Superior orbital fissure
16. Oblique orbital line
17. Orbital process of zygoma

Figure 2B is a skull preparation in the Caldwell position for comparison.

Figure 2C is an anterior pleurodirectional tomogram to show the crista galli (C) and the ethmoidal sinus roof (E). The cribriform plate lies between these structures. Inflammatory mucous membrane thickening partly opacifies the right maxillary sinus.

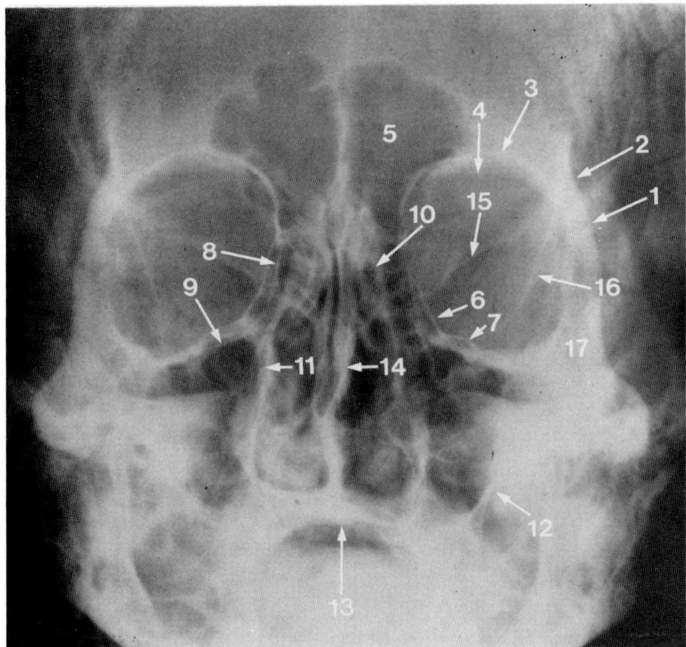

Figure 2A. Caldwell view. See text for key.

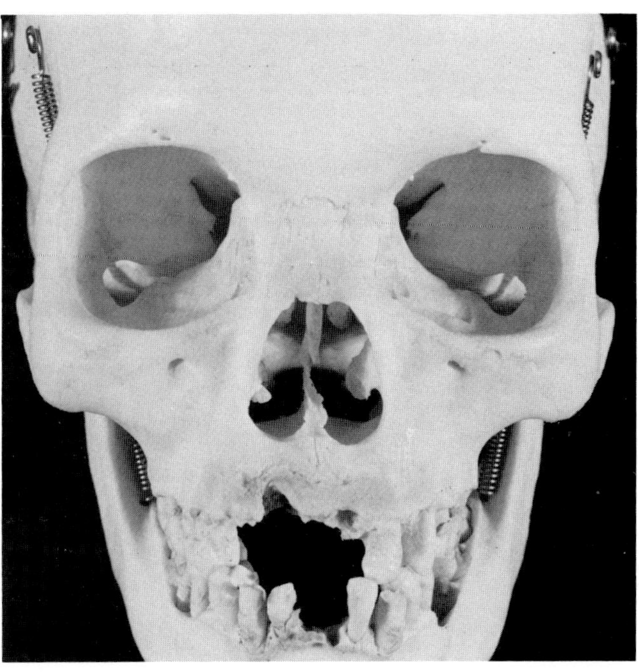

Figure 2B. Skull in Caldwell position.

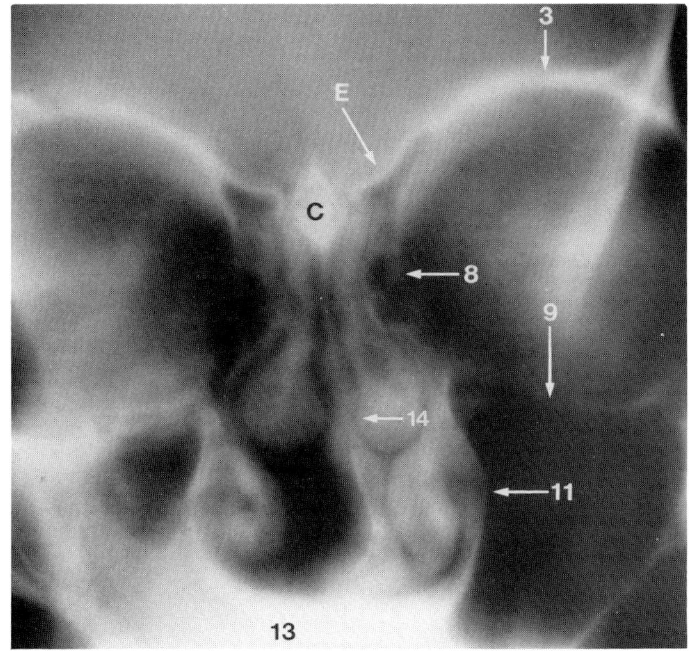

Figure 2C. Anterior coronal tomogram showing the crista galli (C) and ethmoidal sinus roof-fovea ethmoidalis (E). See key in text for numbered structures.

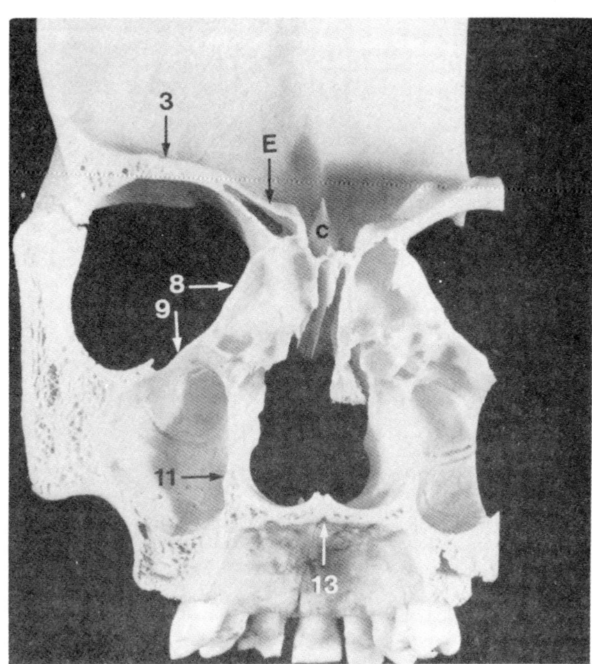

Figure 2D. Companion skull preparation same key as Figure 2C.

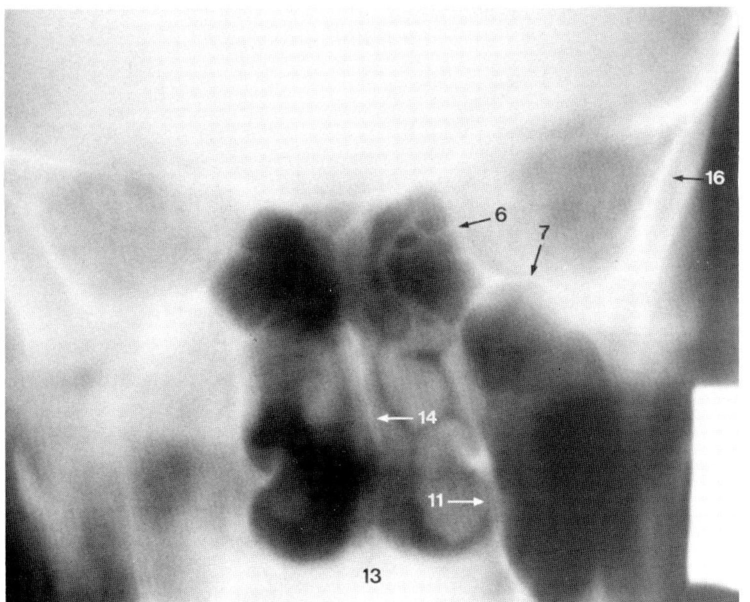

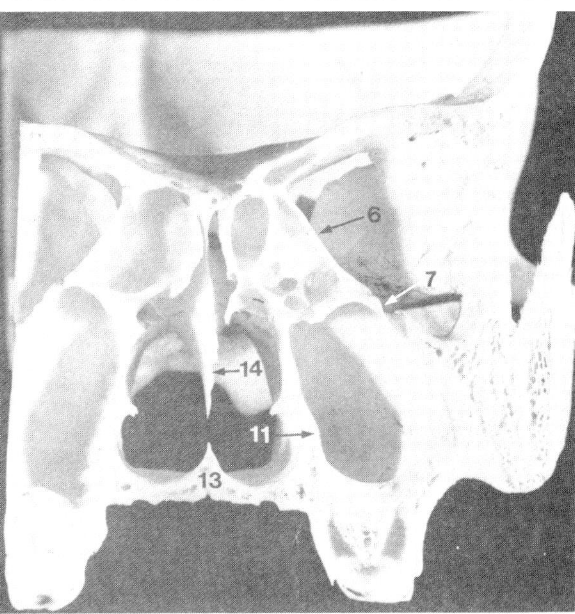

Figure 2E. Posterior coronal tomogram to show continuity of the lamina papyracea and the posterior orbital floor. See key in text for numbered structures.

Figure 2F. Companion skull preparation same key as Figure 2E.

A tomogram at 2 cm more posterior is shown in Figure 2E. This illustrates the relation between the lamina papyracea and the posterior orbital floor.

B. The Waters (Occipitomental) View

The Waters projection uses an occipitomental central ray with the nose and chin against the film holder. The maxillary sinuses are projected above the petrous ridges. The entire zygomatic arch is visible if the view is obtained as a posteroanterior projection.

We do not recommend tomography in this position since the main horizontal facial features—the maxillary alveolus, orbital floor, and roof—are no longer perpendicular to the tomographic plane and may not be sharply visible as they are in the Caldwell position.

The following list of anatomic features is given in a suggested study sequence for Figure 3A. (Numbers are the same as above. Features not visible on this view are omitted).

    1. Zygomaticofrontal suture
    2. Orbital process of frontal bone
    4. Upper (palpable) orbital rim
    5. Frontal sinus
    6. Lamina papyracea
    7. Posterior orbital floor
  12. Lateral maxillary wall
  13. Hard palate
  18. Glenoid fossa of temporomandibular joint
  19. Upper zygomatic arch margin
  20. Lower zygomatic arch margin

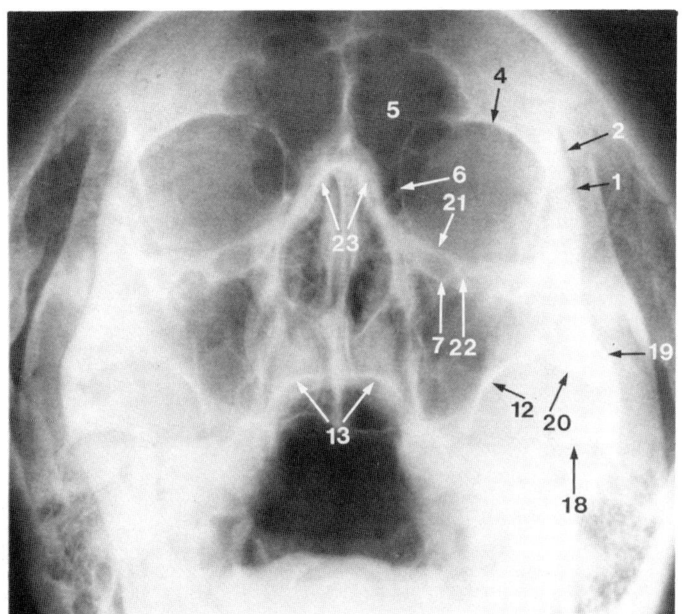

Figure 3A. Waters view. See text for key.

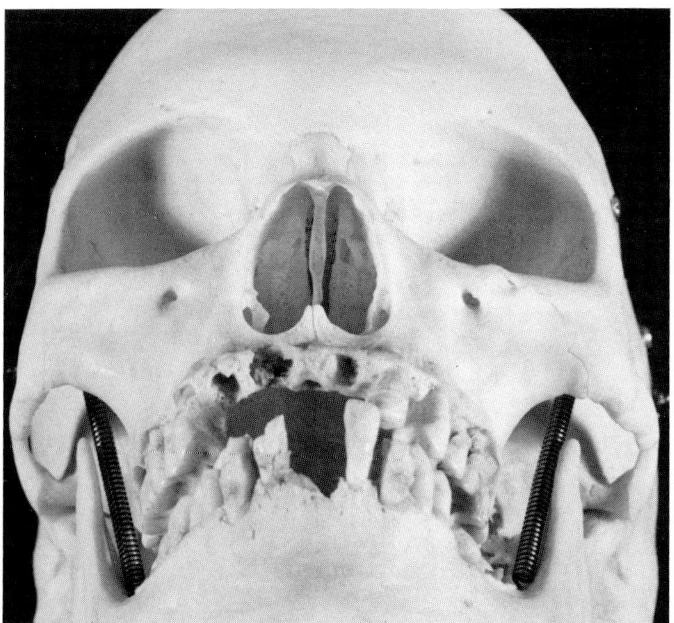

Figure 3B. Skull in Waters position.

21. Lower palpable orbital rim
22. Infraorbital foramen
23. Nasal arch

If one connects the outer border of the orbit (1 and 2) with the upper border of the zygoma (19) and the glenoid fossa (18), and then draws in the lower zygomatic arch (20) and lateral maxillary wall (12), the lines will outline the shape of an elephant head. The orbital processes are the forehead, the zygoma is the trunk, and the lateral maxillary wall is the chin. If this is done on the numbered side of Figure 3A (readers right side), the elephant is looking toward the readers right. The opposite side faces the other way. Our radiology residents have found this to be a helpful way of assessing the integrity of the area. There should be no interruption or asymmetry of the elephant head on either side.

Figure 3B is a view of the skull in Waters position.

C. The Lateral View

In the plain lateral view, structures on the two sides tend to overlap and obscure one another. The sella is well visualized and serves as a guide to the planum sphenoidale (roof of the sphenoid). The planum (A) and hard palate nasal surface (B) should be parallel to each other. An imaginary perpendicular line connecting the frontal sinus anterior surface, anterior nasal spine, and mandible symphysis (C) should parallel a perpendicular line along the greater sphenoidal wing and posterior maxilla (D).

These relationships help define facial bone position on the lateral view. Figure 4 illustrates these relationships.

The lateral position is the other major tomographic projection for evaluating facial injury.

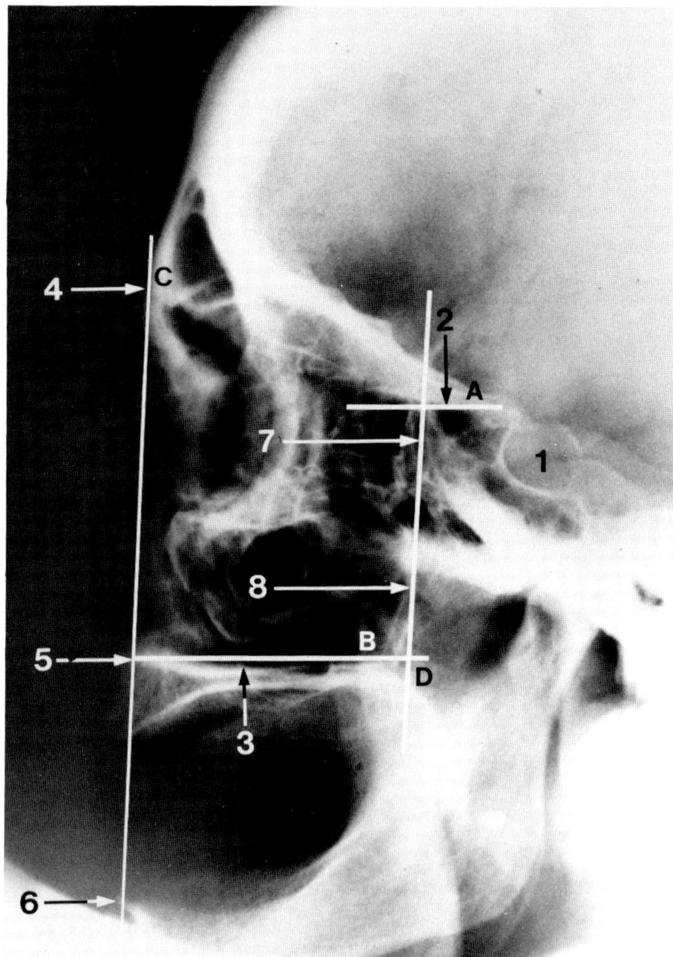

Figure 4. Lateral view 1. Sella. 2. Planum sphenoidale (A). 3. Nasal surface of hard palate (B). 4. Frontal sinus surface. 5. Anterior nasal spine. 6. Symphysis of mandible (C = 4,5 and 6). 7. Greater sphenoidal wing. 8. Posterior maxillary wall (D = 7 and 8).

Figure 5A is a lateral tomogram of the zygomatic recess of the maxillary sinus and zygomatic and frontal process of the lateral orbital wall. A companion view of the skull is shown in Figure 5B.

The lateral orbital wall is more completely seen in Figure 5C. In this, the orbital roof and sphenoidal wing are seen in section as is the zygomatic recess of the maxillary sinus. The zygomaticofrontal and zygomaticosphenoidal suture can be followed from the lateral orbital border to the inferior orbital fissure.

A midorbit tomogram is illustrated by Figure 5D. The fused maxillary posterior wall and pterygoid process are well seen. Figure 5E is a companion skull preparation.

Figure 5F is a midline tomogram. The position is best defined by the sella. The frontal sinus surfaces are well visualized. The palatal horizontal buttress and the perpendicular vomer are also well shown in this view.

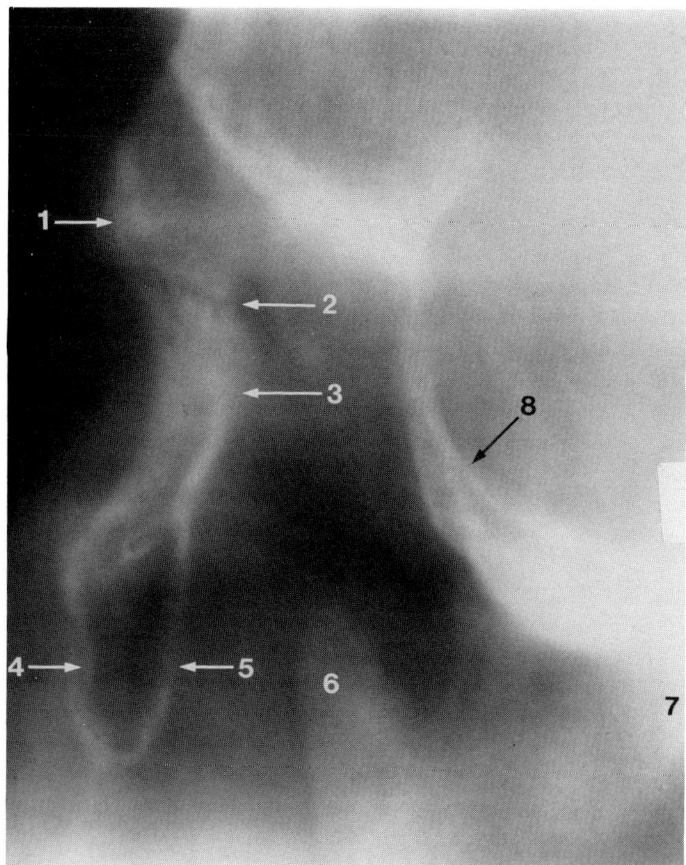

Figure 5A. Lateral tomogram in zygomatico-frontal plane. 1. Frontal process of orbit. 2. Zygomaticofrontal suture. 3. Zygomatic process of orbit. 4. Anterior surface zygomatic recess of maxilla. 5. Posterior wall of zygomatic recess. 6. Coronoid process of mandible. 7. Mandibular condyle. 8. Greater sphenoidal wing.

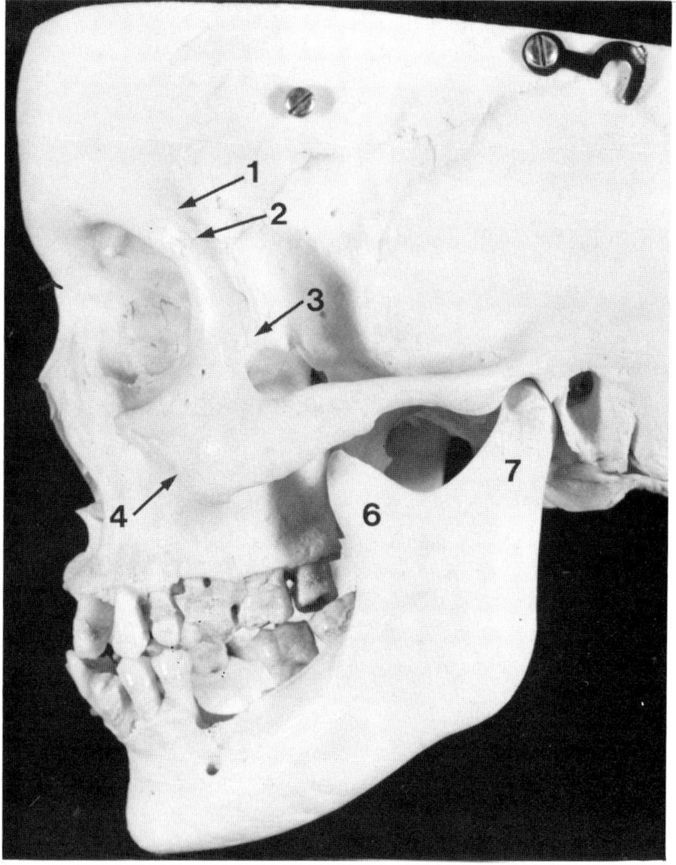

Figure 5B. Companion skull preparation. Key same as Figure 5A.

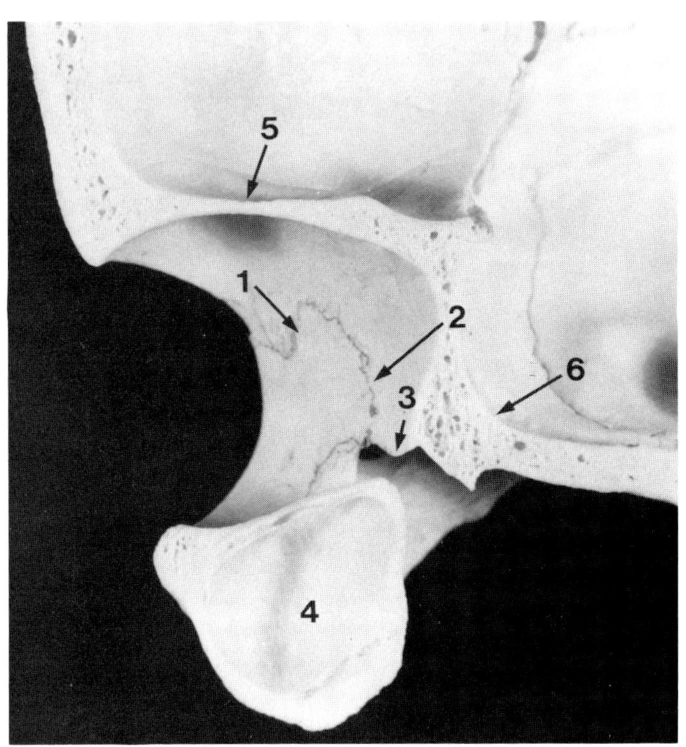

Figure 5C. Section through the outer one-third of the orbit to show the lateral orbital wall. 1. Zygomaticofrontal suture. 2. Zygomaticosphenoidal suture 3. Inferior orbital fissure. 4. Zygomatic recess of maxillary sinus. 5. Orbital roof. 6. Greater sphenoidal wing.

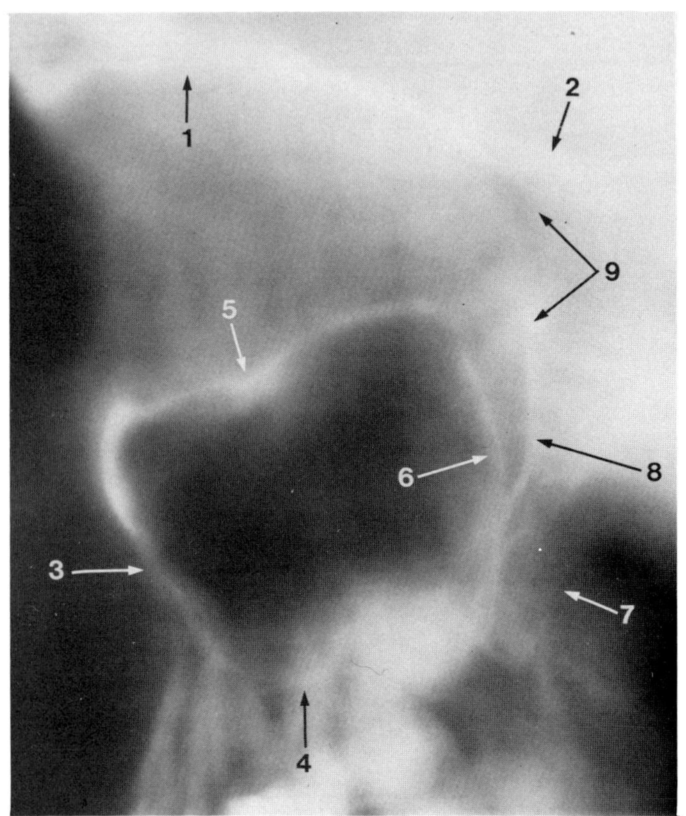

Figure 5D. Midorbit tomogram. 1. Orbital roof. 2. Lesser sphenoidal wing—anterior clinoid process. 3. Anterior maxillary wall. 4. Alveolus. 5. Orbital floor (maxillary roof). 6. Posterior maxillary wall. 7. Pterygoid process. 8. Pterygomaxillary fossa. 9. Superior orbital fissure.

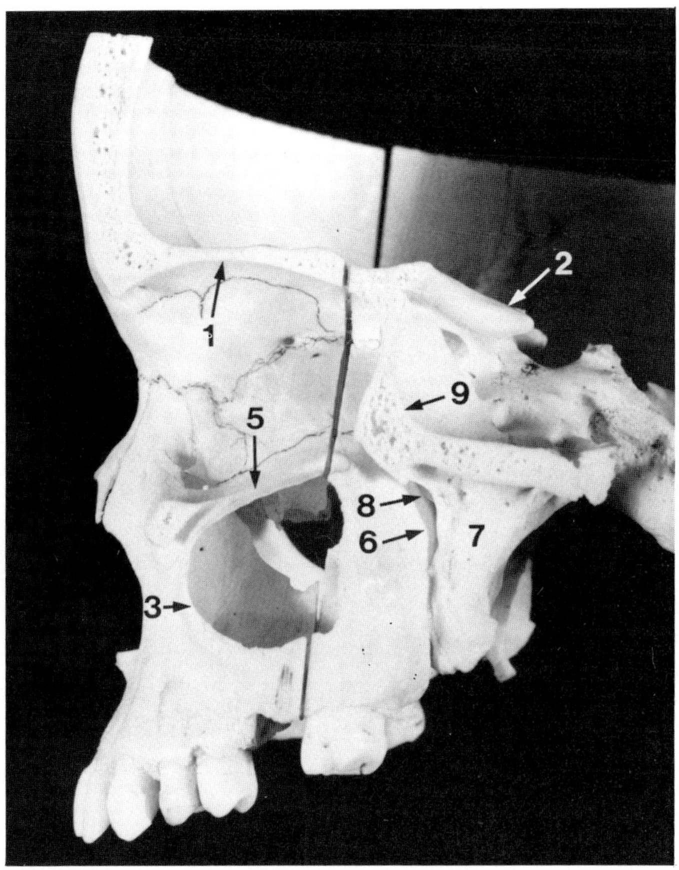

Figure 5E. Midorbit skull preparation. Key same as Figure 5D.

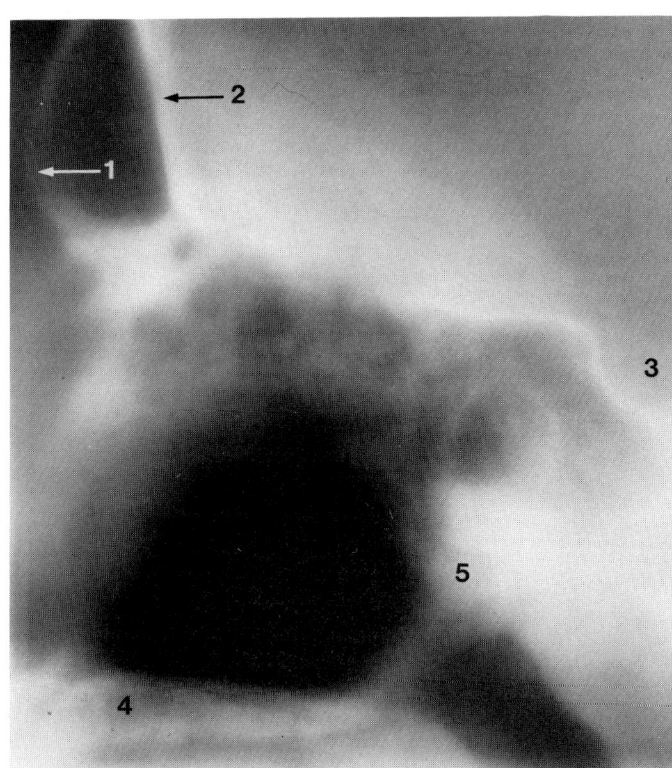

Figure 5F. Midline lateral tomogram. 1. Anterior frontal sinus wall. 2. Posterior frontal sinus wall. 3. Sella turcica. 4. Hard palate. 5. Vomer.

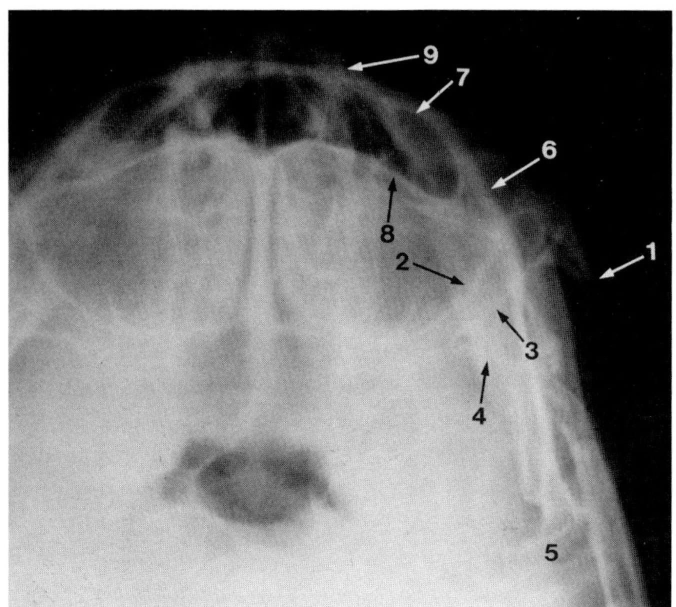

Figure 6A. Basal view. 1. Zygomatic arch. 2. Lateral maxillary sinus wall. 3. Lateral orbit wall. 4. Greater wing of sphenoid. 5. Mandibular condyle. 6. Horizontal mandibular ramus. 7. Anterior frontal sinus wall. 8. Posterior frontal sinus wall. 9. Lateral nasal fossa.

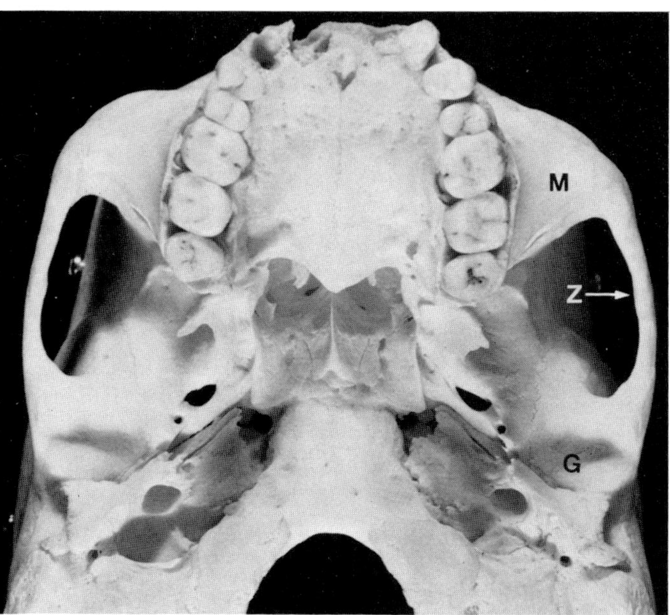

Figure 6B. Skull in basal position to show the glenoid fossa (G), Zygomatic arch (Z), and the maxilla (M).

D. The Basal View

The submental vertex position is of value in assessing the zygomatic arches and mandible, but may not be obtainable in the case of severe facial injury.

Information about the frontal sinus walls, the lateral orbit, the lateral maxillary sinus wall, and the greater sphenoid wing may also be obtained. In the edentulous patient, one may also see the lateral margins of the nasal fossa.

Figure 6A illustrates these features in a basal (submental vertex) projection.

Figure 6B is a skull preparation in the basal position to show the zygomatic arch continuity between the temporal and maxillary extremities.

3. CT ANATOMY

A. Axial CT

The basal tomographic examination shows the same structures as the axial CT views. We customarily obtain layers 0.5-cm thick and in contiguous planes beginning at the maxillary alveolus level and continuing through the frontal sinus area. These views best illustrate the perpendicular buttresses of facial structures. The CT examining plane should show horizontal structures also, but frequently is slightly oblique so that the hard palate, zygomatic arch, orbital floor, and roof may only be seen in part on a given section.

Anatomic structures present in the four principal axial CT planes are illustrated.

Figure 7A is located in the plane of the dental alveolus. A maxillary retention cyst produces opacity on the readers left. Maxillary sinus detail is most evident on the midmaxillary plane in Figure 7B. This view is 16 mm above that shown in Figure 7A.

The third principal CT plane is at the level of the orbital floor. This plane represents the major horizontal portion of the midface. The entire zygomatic arch may be seen. The posterior maxillary sinus air cell extends upward as seen in the lateral view of the midorbit. The nasal bone and the frontal process of the maxilla are now evident anteriorly. The anterior and posterior lacrimal crests enclose the lacrimal fossa along the medial orbital border. These features are seen in Figure 7C.

The highest principal CT plane passes through the center of the orbit, the ethmoidal, and the sphenoidal sinuses. The zygomatic and sphenoidal orbital processes form the lateral wall that connects posteriorly to the greater sphenoidal wing. Figure 7D illustrates these features.

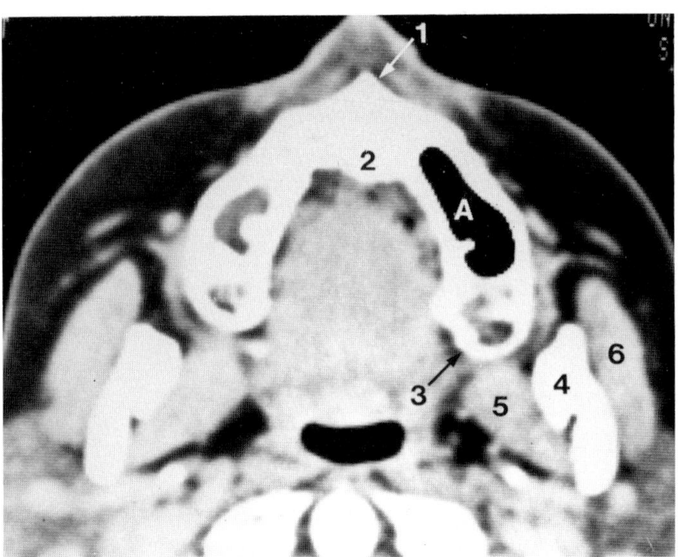

Figure 7A. Axial CT of maxillary alveolus (A). 1. Anterior nasal spine. 2. Anterior hard palate. 3. Maxillary tuberosity. 4. Vertical ramus of mandible. 5. Medial pterygoid muscle. 6. Masseter muscle.

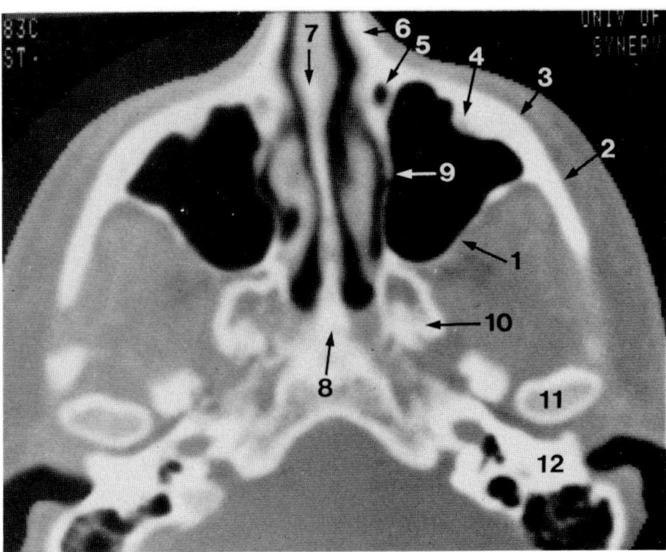

Figure 7B. Midmaxillary plane on axial CT. 1. Lateral maxillary wall. 2. Anterior zygomatic arch. 3. Anterior maxillary surface. 4. Section of infraorbital canal. 5. Bony canal for lacrimal duct. 6. Nasal pyramidal (frontal) process of maxilla. 7. Perpendicular ethmoidal plate. 8. Vomer. 9. Medial maxillary wall. 10. Pterygoid process. 11. Mandibular condyle. 12. Tympanic surface of temporomandibular joint.

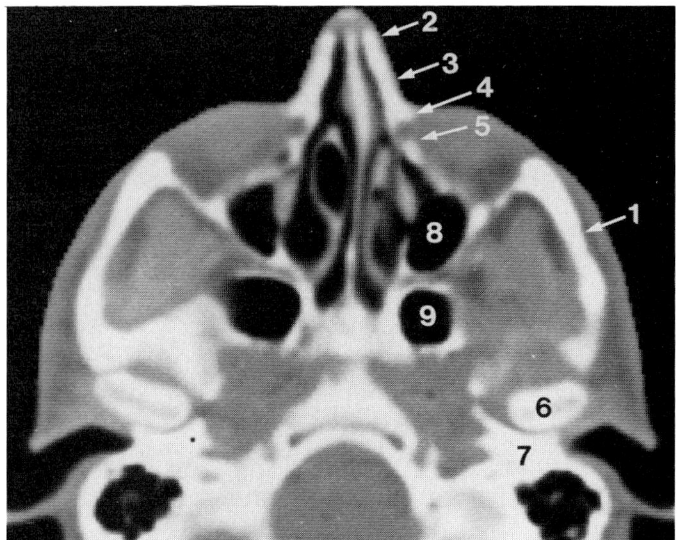

Figure 7C. Axial CT in plane of orbital floor. 1. Zygomatic arch. 2. Nasal bone. 3. Frontal process of maxilla. 4. Anterior lacrimal crest. 5. Posterior lacrimal crest. 6. Mandibular condyle. 7. Tympanic bone. 8. Upper maxillary sinus. 9. Sphenoidal sinus cell in base of pterygoid process.

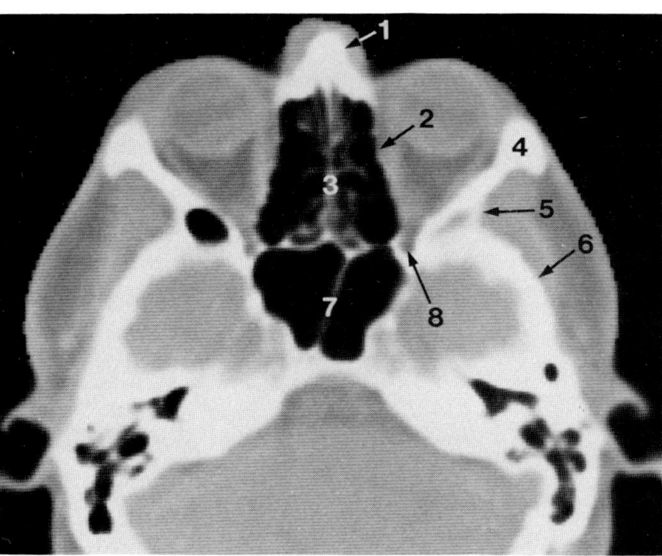

Figure 7D. Midorbit on axial CT. 1. Glabella. 2. Lamina papyracea. 3. Ethmoidal sinus cell complex. 4. Zygomatic portion of lateral orbit. 5. Sphenoidal process of lateral orbital wall. 6. Greater wing. 7. Sphenoidal sinus. 8. Superior orbital fissure.

B. Coronal CT

We obtain contiguous, direct coronal slices of 5-mm thickness beginning at the frontal sinus surface and continuing backward to the sella turcica.

Six principal coronal planes are found. The first plane, Figure 8A, is through the frontal sinus and anterior cranial fossa.

The next plane is through the anterior orbital roof, the globe, and frontal process of the maxilla. This plane is illustrated in Figure 8B.

The midorbital plane is through the center of the globe and includes the entire orbit wall, the anterior portion of the ethmoidal sinuses, and the anterior maxillary sinuses. Figure 8C illustrates the midorbital plane.

The retrobulbar plane is behind the eye and reveals the optic nerve and rectus muscles if printed as a soft tissue representation as shown in Figure 8D. The ethmoid and maxillary sinus walls are well defined as is the inferior nasal turbinate and hard palate.

The superior and inferior orbital fissures are the main landmarks of the next coronal plane as seen in Figure 8E. Posterior ethmoid and maxillary sinus spaces surround the nasal fossa where the inferior, middle, and superior turbinates are located. The superior orbital fissure lies just lateral to the ethmoid sinus and communicates with the inferior orbital fissure that is located just above the posterior maxillary sinus. A thin layer of the posterior frontal bone encloses the top of the superior fissure.

The last coronal CT plane is through the level of the choana and the pterygoid plates of the sphenoid bone. Figure 8F shows the relation between the greater wing and the pterygoid processes and how the posterior buttresses merge with the posterior palate.

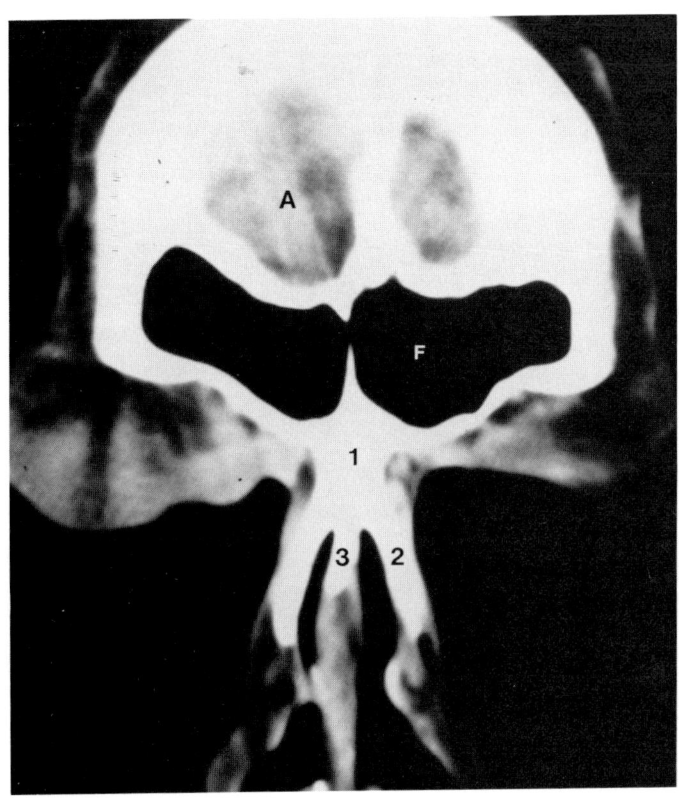

Figure 8A. Anterior plane through the frontal sinus. A. Anterior cranial fossa. F. Frontal sinus. 1. Glabella. 2. Nasal arch. 3. Perpendicular plate of the ethmoid bone.

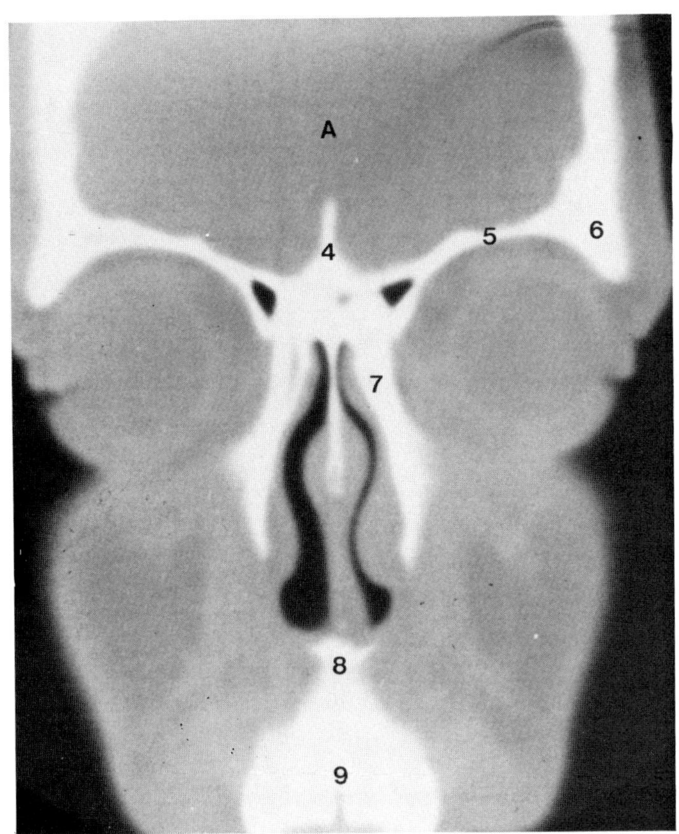

Figure 8B. Anterior orbit roof, globe, and frontal process of maxilla plane. A. Anterior cranial fossa. 4. Crista galli. 5. Anterior orbital roof. 6. Orbital process of frontal bone. 7. Orbital process of maxilla. 8. Anterior nasal spine. 9. Central and lateral teeth.

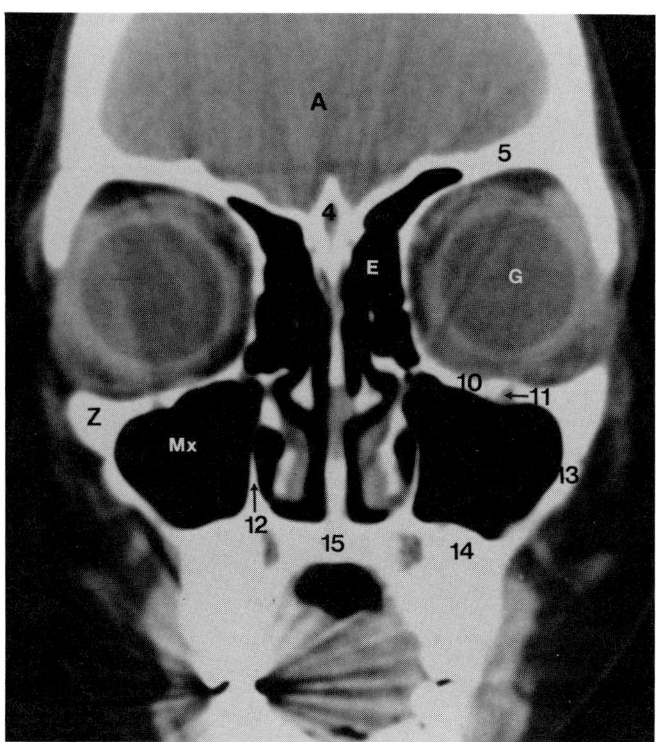

Figure 8C. Midorbit plane. A. Anterior fossa. G. Globe. 4. Crista galli. 5. Anterior orbital roof. E. Ethmoidal sinus (with supraorbital recess). 10. Orbital floor. 11. Infraorbital canal. Z. Zygoma. Mx. Maxillary sinus. 12. Medial maxillary wall. 13. Lateral maxillary wall. 14. Maxillary alveolus. 15. Hard palate and vomer.

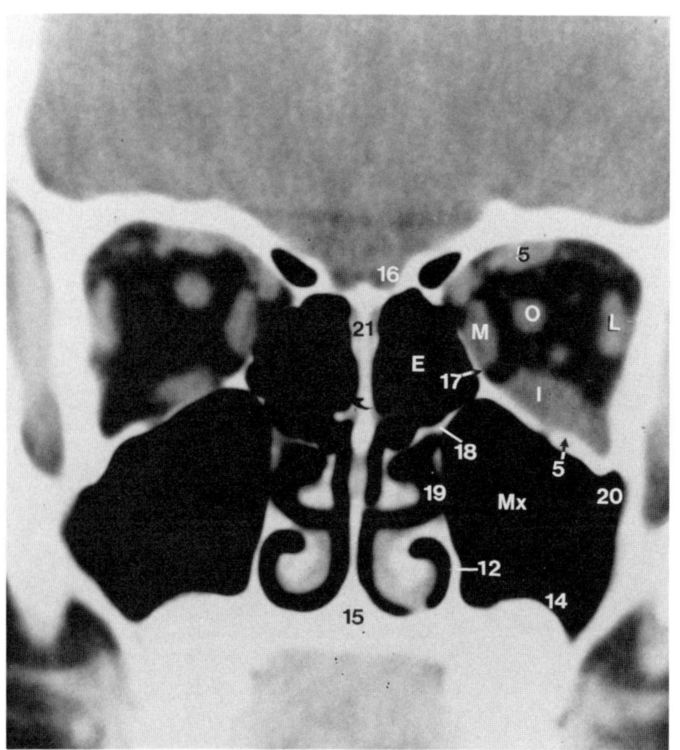

Figure 8D. Retrobulbar plane. Orbital soft tissues. O. Optic nerve. S. Superior rectus and levator palpebre muscles. L. Lateral rectus muscle. M. Medial rectus muscle. I. Inferior rectus muscle. E. Ethmoidal sinus. 16. Ethmoid roof. 17. Lamina papyracea. 18. Ethmoid-maxillary sinus septum. Mx. Maxillary sinus. 5. Maxillary roof (orbit floor). 19. Sinus ostium. 12. Medial maxillary wall. 14. Alveolar recess. 20. Zygomatic recess. 15. Hard palate. 21. Perpendicular plate of the ethmoid.

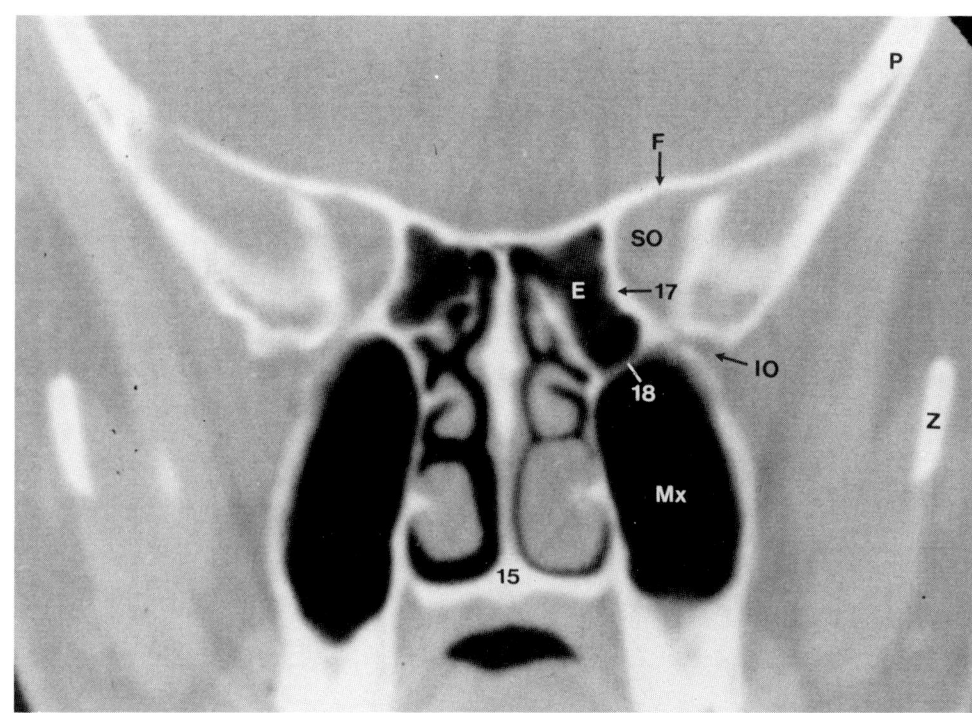

Figure 8E. Superior and inferior orbital fissure plane. SO. Superior orbital fissure. IO. Inferior orbital fissure. E. Ethmoidal sinus. 17. Lamina papyracea. F. Frontal bone. 18. Maxillary-ethmoid septum. Mx. Maxillary sinus. 15. Hard palate and vomer. Z. Zygomatic arch. P. Pteryion.

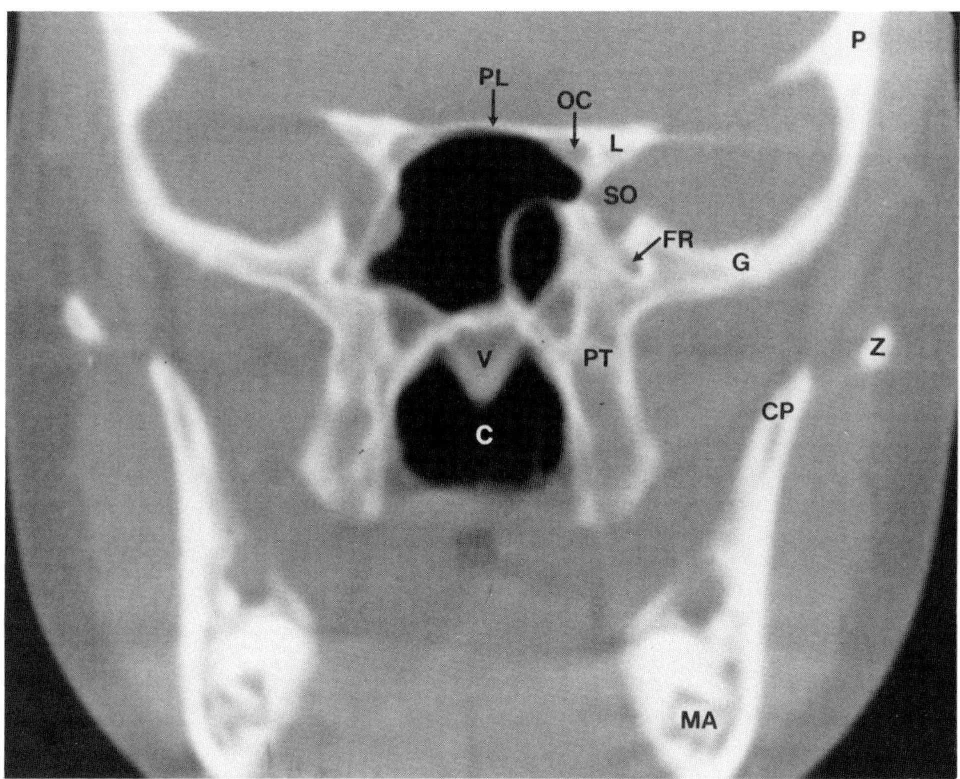

Figure 8F. Plane of the choana and pterygoid plates. PL. Planum sphenoidale. L. Lesser wing of sphenoid. OC. Optic canal. SO. Superior orbital fissure. FR. Foramen rotundum. G. Greater wing of sphenoid. PT. Pterygoid plates. V. Vomer. C. Choanae. P. Pteryion. Z. Zygomatic arches. CP. Coronoid process. MA. Mandible angle.

4. SPECIAL CONSIDERATIONS ABOUT THE ORBIT AND EYE

A. The Oblique Orbital Line

The oblique orbital line (OOL) is produced by the orbital process of the sphenoid, which contributes to the lateral orbital wall. This process is well visualized on the midorbit axial CT plane (Figure 7D). The OOL is also present in the Caldwell (Figure 2A) and Waters (Figure 3A) views.

Figure 9 is an anterior facial skeleton preparation in which drill cuts are used to define different parts of the lateral orbital wall. Cut 1 is through the orbital process of the zygoma posterior to the zygomaticofrontal suture. This cut lies lateral to the OOL.

Cut 2 is through the orbital process of the sphenoid and interrupts the OOL. If this cut is continued further posteriorly into the greater wing proper, the lucent line extends through the OOL. and both medially and laterally into the greater wing proper as seen in cut 3.

Surgical confirmation of what the OOL represents is found in Figures 10A and 10B. The Naquin-Reece lateral orbitotomy is a procedure whereby the surgeon gains access to retrobulbar structures through a resection of the thin sphenoidal and zygomatic processes of the lateral orbital wall. Following this resection, the OOL disappears as seen in Figure 10A.

The Kronlein procedure is another orbitotomy procedure in which the entire lateral orbital wall is removed back to the greater wing. This type of resection also removes the OOL, as demonstrated by Figure 10B. Since we already know the orbital process of the zygoma does not produce the OOL (Figure 9), the orbital process of the sphenoid must produce this line.

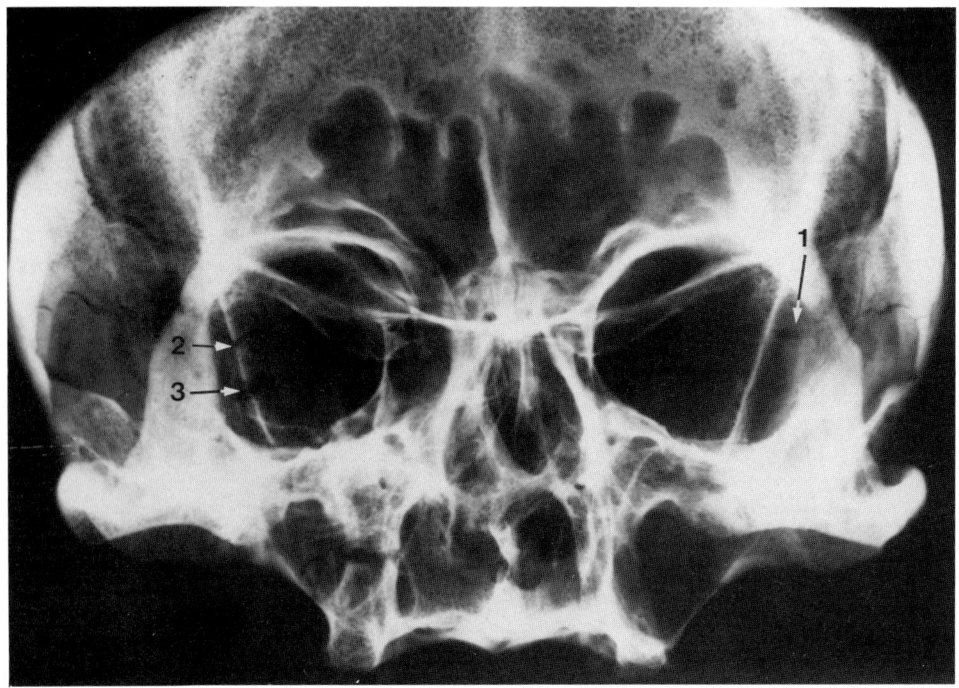

Figure 9. Anterior facial skeleton preparation. 1. Drill cut through orbital process of zygoma. 2. Cut through orbital process of sphenoid. 3. Posterior continuation of cut 2.

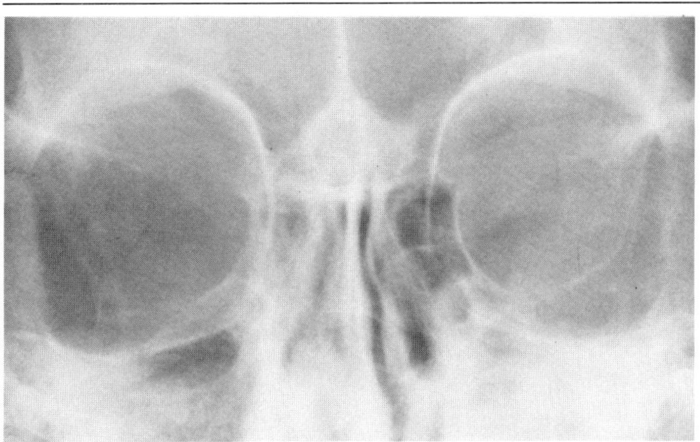

Figure 10A. The OOL following surgery. Caldwell view after a right Naquin-Reece orbitotomy. The OOL is missing.

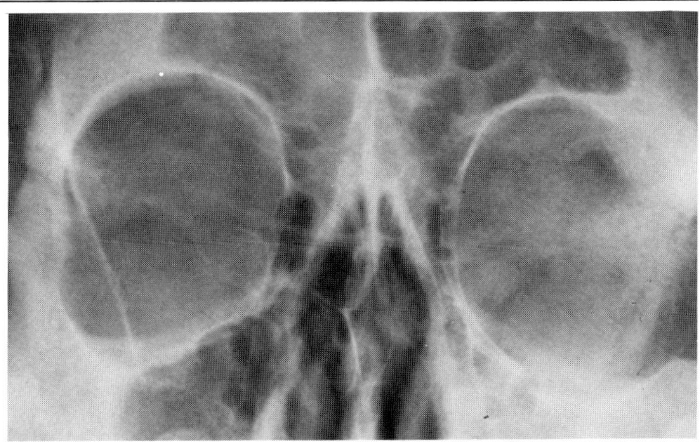

Figure 10B. Caldwell view showing absent left OOL after Kronlein orbitotomy.

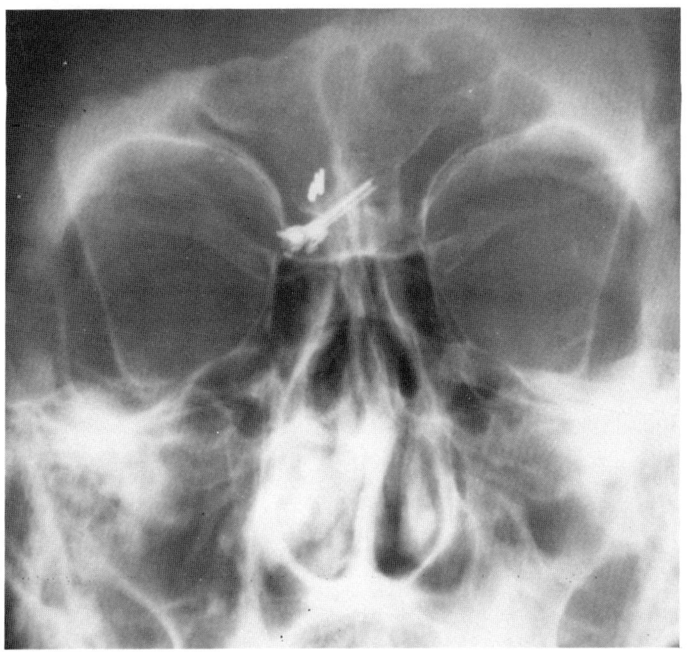

Figure 10C. Caldwell view after right frontal and anterior sphenoidal wing resection for aneurysm. The OOL is present.

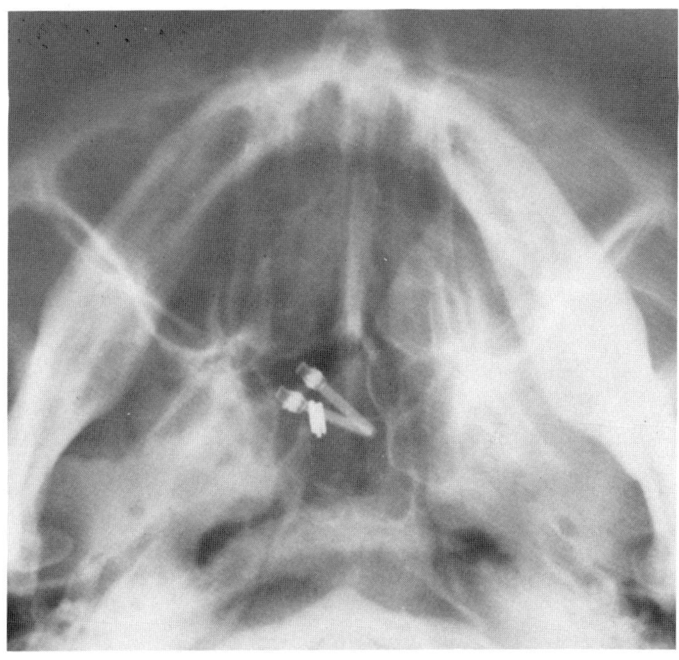

Figure 10D. Basal view with resection of part of the greater wing on the right.

Some authors have attributed the OOL to a portion of the greater sphenoid wing peripheral to the orbital process. Again, surgical evidence refutes this idea. The Caldwell view in Figure 10C demonstrates a large craniotomy, involving the right frontal bone and greater wing, which was made to allow the surgeon to place a clip on a carotid aneurysm. The sphenoidal portion of this flap extended to the edge of the orbital process as seen in the basal view illustrated by Figure 10D. Yet the OOL is clearly defined on the Caldwell view.

The following examples show how information regarding the OOL can be used in fracture analysis.

A patient with a slightly displaced left tripod fracture, not clearly shown on the Caldwell view in Figure 11A, also has interruption of the caudal OOL. This allows one to see the transverse fracture extending into the superior orbital fissure.

Figure 11B is a Waters view of a patient with an extensive frontal sinus anterior wall and upper orbital rim fracture on the right (poorly seen). The right OOL is interrupted, thus suggesting extension of the frontal fracture across the orbital roof. This was confirmed by tomography.

The patient, illustrated by the Waters view in Figure 11C, has a right tripod fracture and an interrupted OOL. Lateral to the OOL separation, one can follow the fracture that extends posterolaterally into the temporal fossa.

Avulsion of the right zygoma and orbital process of the sphenoid without a fracture of the greater wing is illustrated by Figure 11D.

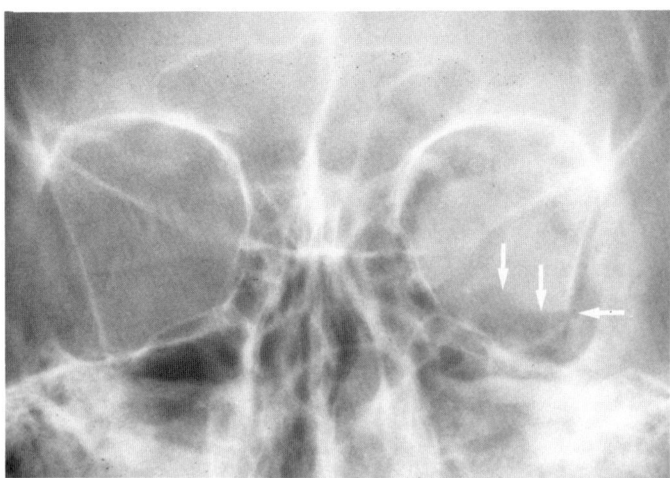

Figure 11A. Fracture analysis of the OOL. Caldwell view with OOL interruption on left at horizontal arrow. Medial extension of fracture into superior fissure at vertical arrows.

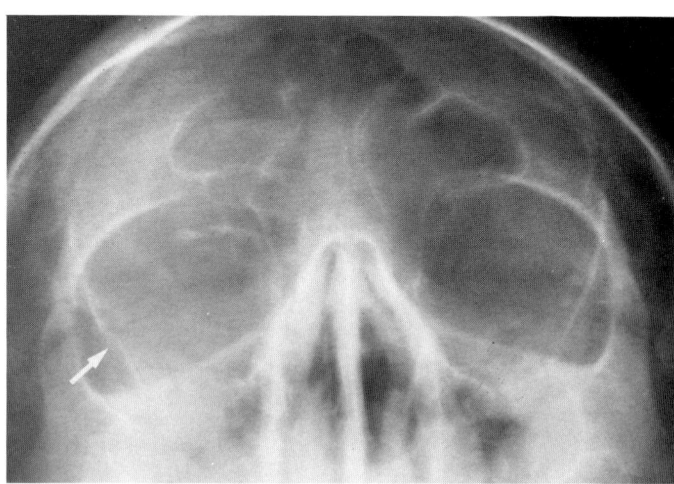

Figure 11B. Frontal sinus and upper orbital rim fracture on right in Waters view. Interrupted right OOL at arrow suggested an orbital roof fracture proved on other views.

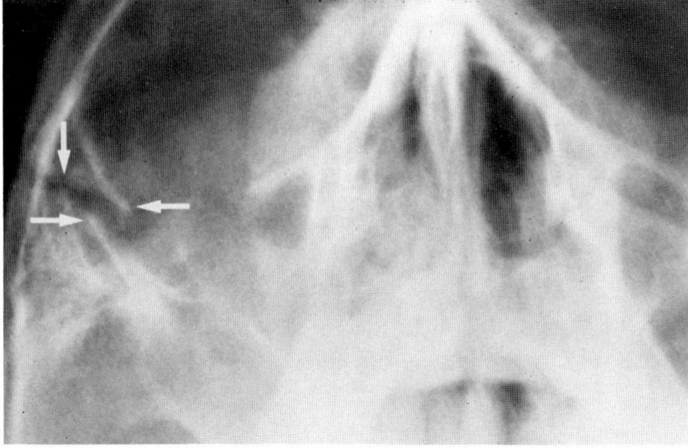

Figure 11C. Interrupted OOL on right at horizontal arrows lead to a greater wing fracture extending laterally at vertical arrow.

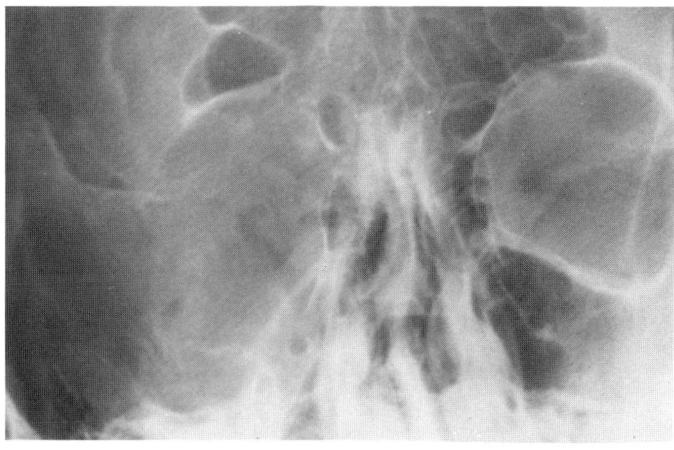

Figure 11D. Caldwell view with complete avulsion of the zygoma and absent right OOL. Greater wing and superior fissure are intact.

These cases show the value of assessing the oblique orbital line as an index to the presence of more extensive injury about the posterolateral portion of the orbit.

B. Soft Tissue Injuries of the Eye

Both periocular and intraocular injuries may occur alone or may be part of and associated with a fracture. One of the signs of injury involving the sinus surfaces of the orbit is the presence of periocular air. This may arise from the ethmoidal sinus most commonly, but frontal and maxillary sinus wall injuries may also result in this change.

Figure 12 illustrates a large bilateral preseptal air accumulation secondary to a nasal-ethmoidal sinus fracture. The air is largely in front of the orbital septum, but two small air bubbles are present posteriorly in the muscle cone. One must be careful in evaluating CT scans not to misinterpret the presence of a small crescentric air accumulation trapped under the eye lid as may occur in patients with no injury. The large volume of air in this case indicates that these are pathological collections.

Preseptal hemorrhage is interposed between the skin surface and the ocular margin on the right side of Figure 13A. This was associated with a tripod fracture accompanied by an ethmoidal fracture that has produced opacity of several adjacent ethmoidal sinus cells.

A higher CT cut in the examination of this patient shows extensive intraocular hemorrhage as well. Figure 13B is an axial CT that shows preseptal

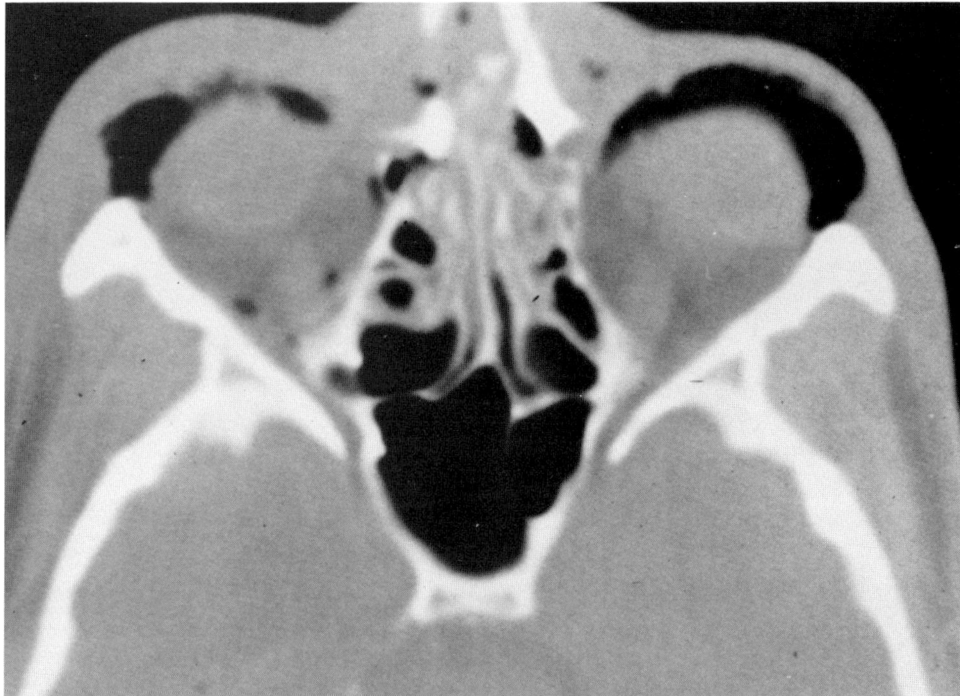

Figure 12. Axial CT scan with large preseptal air accumulations associated with a nasal-ethmoidal comminuted fracture.

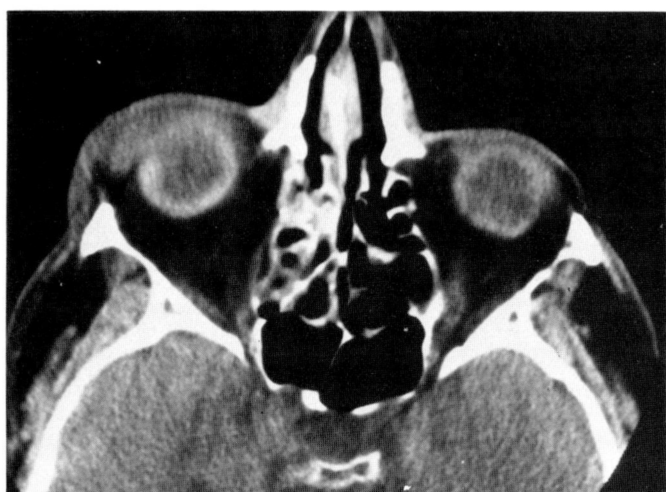

Figure 13A. CT examination of hemorrhage in the preseptal space, vitreous, and retinal surface. An axial CT view showing preseptal blood on the right.

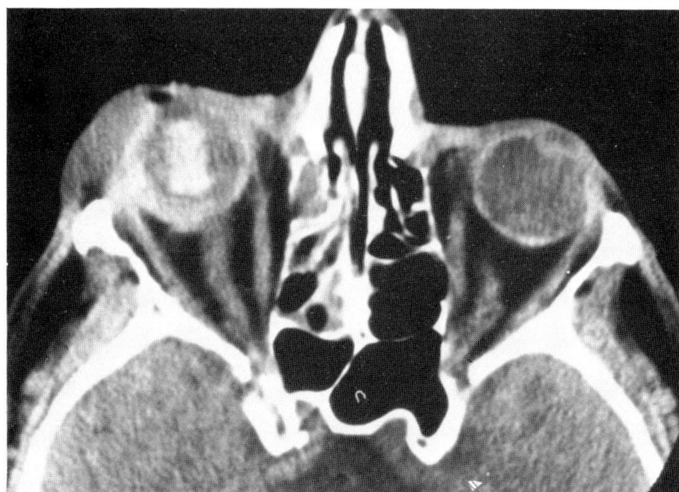

Figure 13B. A higher axial CT cut showing the central vitreous hemorrhage and blood along the lateral retinal surface on the right.

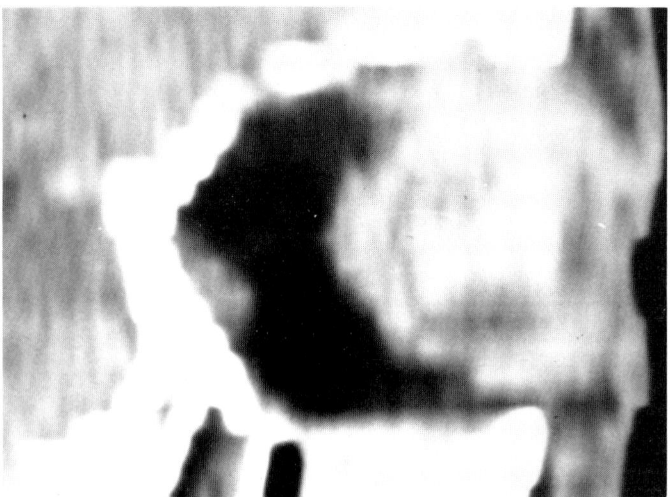

Figure 13C. A lateral CT reconstruction in the same patient.

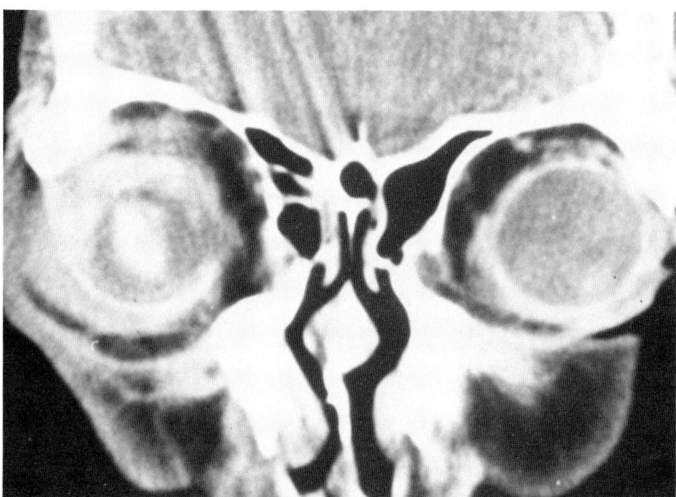

Figure 13D. A direct coronal CT through the midocular plane in the same patient.

hemorrhage and intraocular blood in the vitreous, as well as along the retinal surface of the posterior chamber. The roughly rectangular central increased density area is in the hyaloid canal (Cloquet) and has enlarged the size of the canal. The lens is hidden by the anterior extent of the vitreous blood in this view.

The vitreous blood has a dumbbell shape in the lateral reconstruction illustrated by Figure 13C. A direct coronal CT scan through the middle of the globe, Figure 13D, shows the central vitreous blood, as well as blood over the upper retinal surface.

Lens dislocation is present on the left side along with posterior chamber blood in the patient whose examination is demonstrated by the axial CT in Figure 14. The affected lens has been rotated 90° out of position in comparison to the normal lens position on the right side of this view.

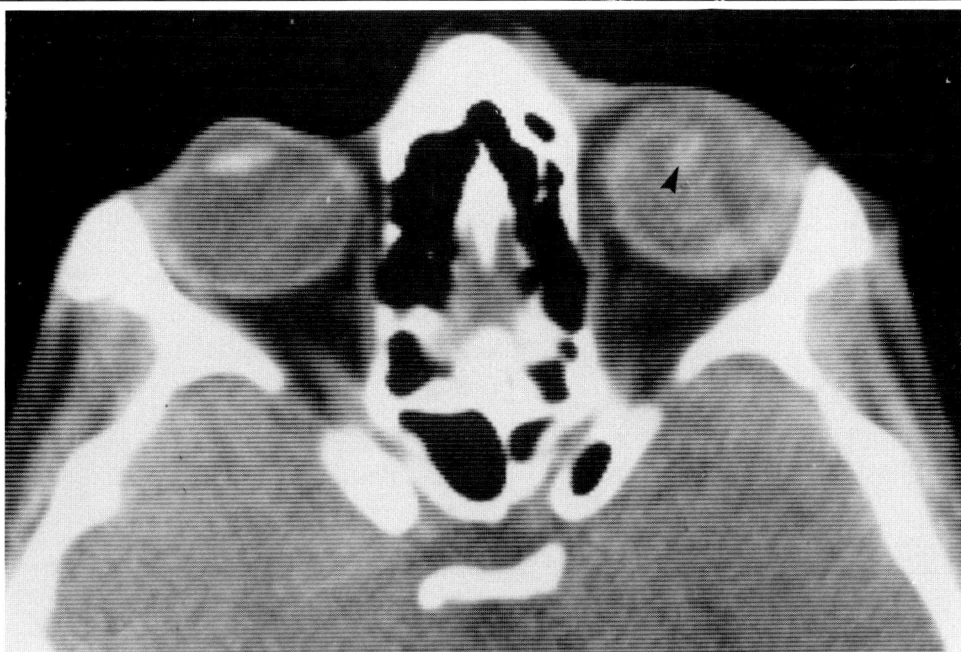

Figure 14. Lens dislocation (arrowhead) in an axial CT examination. Compare this with the normal lens position on the right.

Ocular laceration with a ruptured globe may accompany severe facial skeletal injury as seen in Figure 15 where a completely disorganized left globe reflects the ocular injury. The patient had an extensive fracture of the ethmoidal-frontal axis and the left zygoma. Two air bubbles are in the center of the distorted eye.

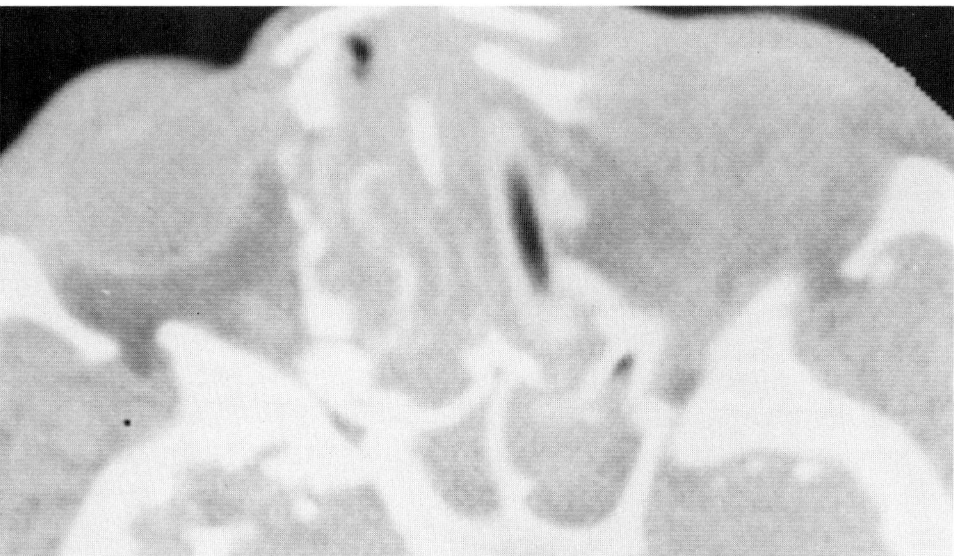

Figure 15. Axial CT with extensive ethmoidal-frontal injury. Ruptured globe on the left with marked distortion.

C. Orbital and Ocular Foreign Bodies

Foreign bodies involving the eye or orbit may occur as a solitary injury or may be associated with facial injury. Radiologic demonstration depends on the density of the foreign material. Usually steel foreign bodies are quite apparent on conventional radiographs. We obtain plain films in the Caldwell projection, one with the patient looking upward and another looking downward to detect movement of an intraocular foreign body. In addition, a lateral view with the injured side placed closest to the film holder is obtained.

Figure 16 illustrates the above examination technique used in a patient with a steel fragment in the right eye. Figure 16A is a view with the patient looking upward. Movement of the foreign body downward in relation to the orbit margin occurs with downward gaze shown in Figure 16B. Since the foreign body moves downward, the object must be in the anterior part of the eye. This position is confirmed by the right lateral view in Figure 16C. If the foreign body is small and located with the rectus muscle or tendon, it

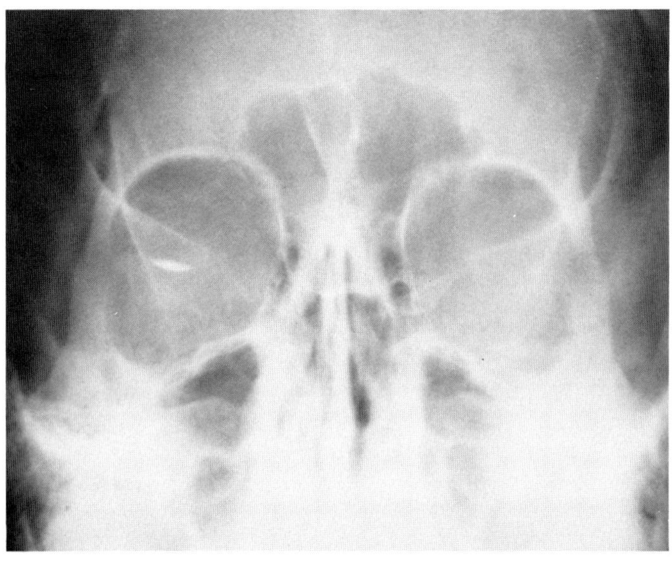

Figure 16A. Metallic foreign body in the right eye. Caldwell view with patient looking upward.

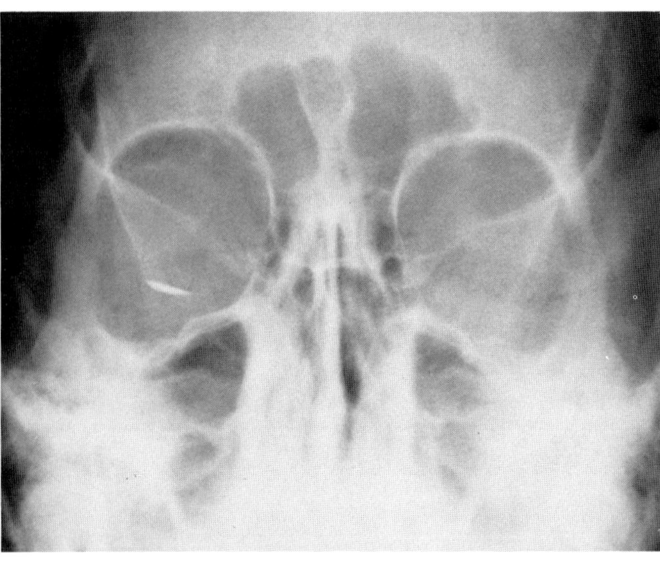

Figure 16B. Same patient. Caldwell view with downward gaze.

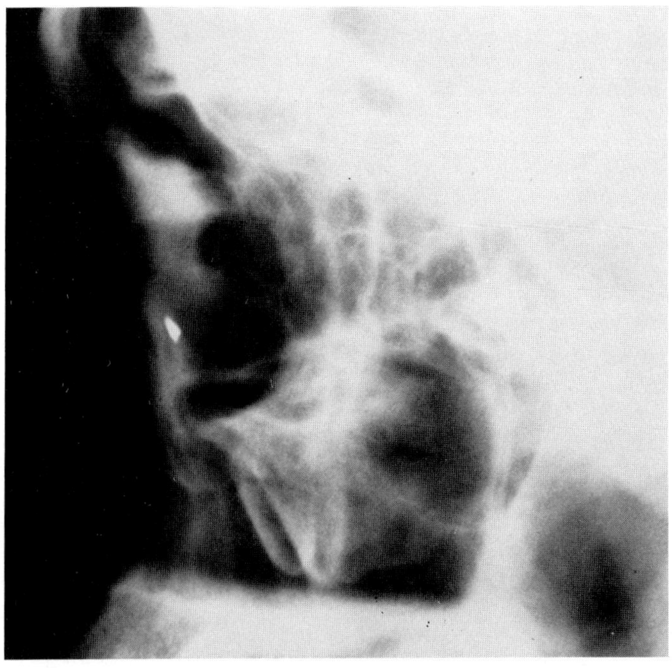

Figure 16C. Same patient. Right lateral view to illustrate the anterior ocular position of the foreign body.

may move as an intraocular foreign body would move. Ultrasound or CT examination may be needed for precise location of a small foreign body.

Large metallic foreign bodies may produce so much artifact on CT examination that localization may be difficult. The Caldwell and lateral plain radiographs in Figures 17A and 17B show a .177-caliber air rifle pellet in the right eye. CT examination in Figure 17C, which is through the center of the pellet, is obscured by subtraction artifacts to such an extent that the intraocular location cannot be established. Subsequent 3-mm axial slices ultimately reach the edge of the foreign body, which produces little artifact,

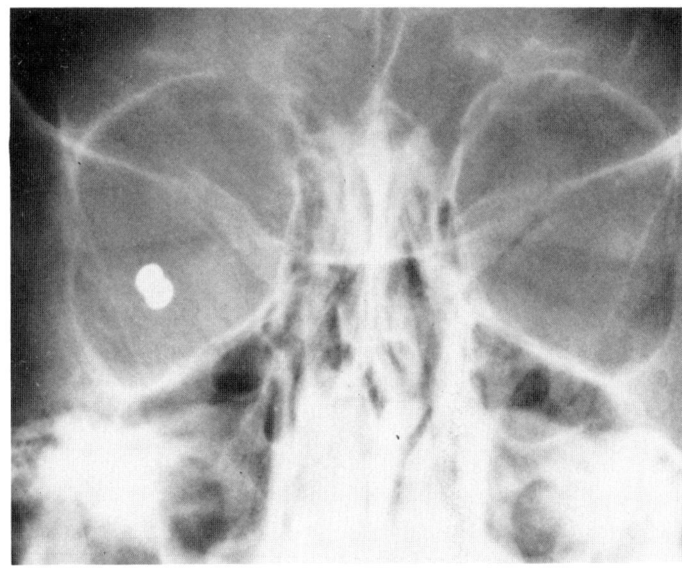

Figure 17A. Patient with a .177-caliber air rifle pellet in the right eye. Waters view.

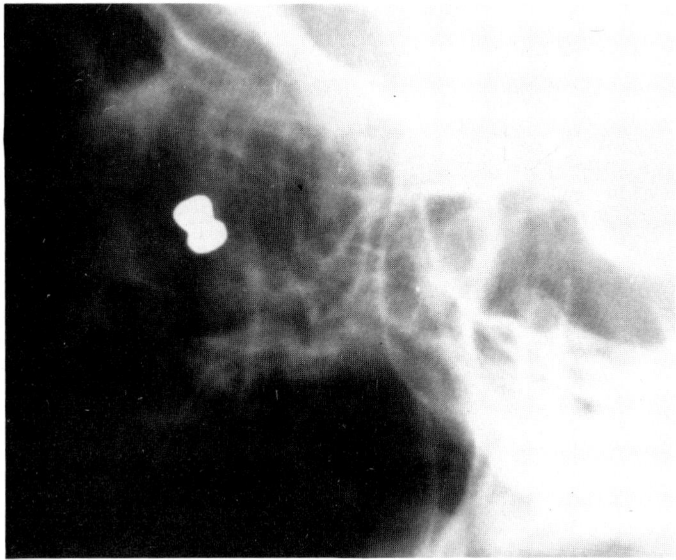

Figure 17B. Same patient. Lateral view.

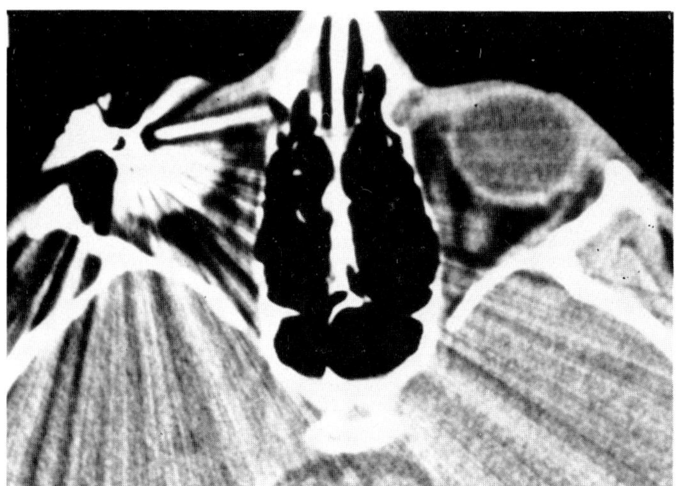

Figure 17C. Same patient. Axial CT with subtraction artifact obscures the location of the foreign body.

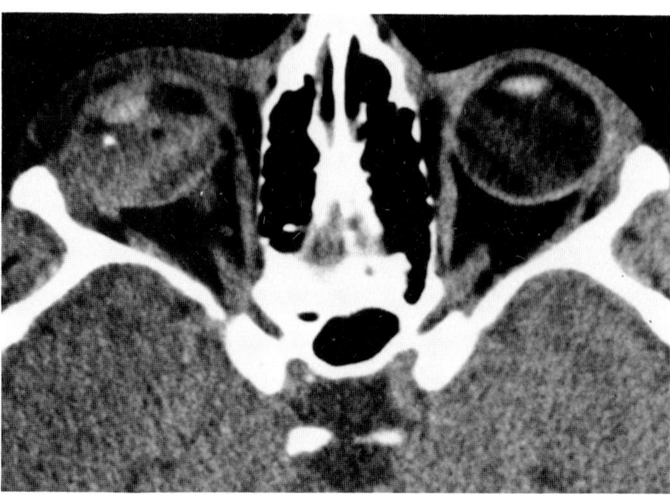

Figure 17D. Same patient. An axial CT at the upper edge of the foreign body shows the foreign body lying in the area of the iris and vitreous. Two intraocular air bubbles are also present.

and show that it lies in the plane of the iris and anterior vitreous. This is demonstrated in Figure 17D in which two ocular air bubbles are also present.

The "edge", or partial volume, effect may give the most reliable anatomic localization of a large metallic foreign body.

Since the average eye is 25 mm in diameter, a 25¢ coin can be used as a rough approximation of the diameter of the eye, since it also is 25 mm in diameter. One may simply center the coin in the frontal and lateral orbital views to determine the foreign body relation to the eye.

Glass used in windshield or bottle construction contains sufficient impurities to be defined on plain films. High-quality glass, such as fine crystal, is radiotransparent. Most plastic, aluminum, and wooden objects are radiotransparent on conventional x-ray films. CT examination may be very helpful in identifying the presence of low-density objects.

Figure 18 is the axial CT examination of a boy who had a wooden stick inserted accidentally into his orbit at a marshmallow roast. The stick was broken off after the injury. Figure 18A is an axial CT through the midorbital

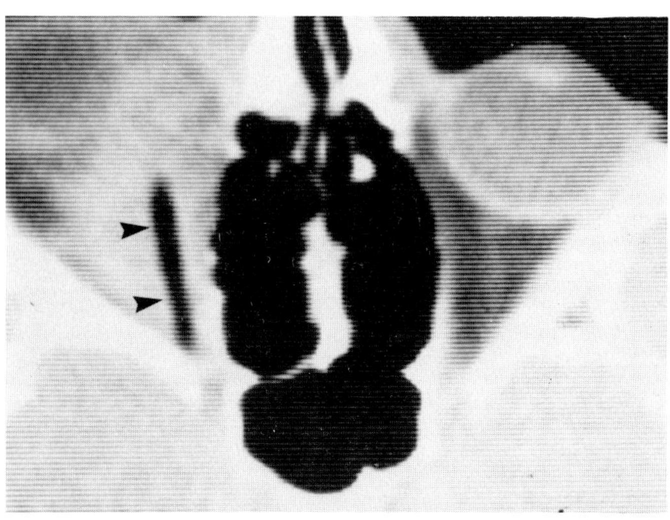

Figure 18A. Wooden foreign body in the orbit. Early axial CT shows a large medial hematoma with a central linear low-density area (arrowheads) representing the stick.

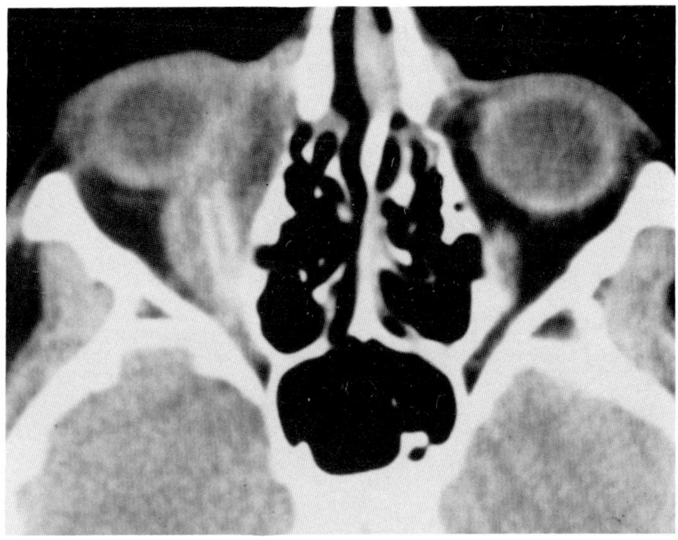

Figure 18B. Same patient. Axial reexamination 2 weeks later shows decrease in the hematoma size and two enhanced lines (arrowheads) representing a residual fragment.

plane. A large perimedian hematoma is present throughout the length of the orbit. In the center of the hematoma is a long black slender object that represents the stick fragment.

Following operative removal of what was thought to be all of the stick, the wound continued to drain suggesting that another part of the stick was still present. Figure 18B is a repeat axial CT examination done 2 weeks after the initial examination. This examination was done with contrast material and shows reduction in size of the hematoma as well as absorption of contrast material by the remaining stick fragment, which produced the two dense lines in the axial view. A coronal reconstruction, Figure 18C, shows a ring of enhancement around the stick fragment which lies along the medial orbit floor.

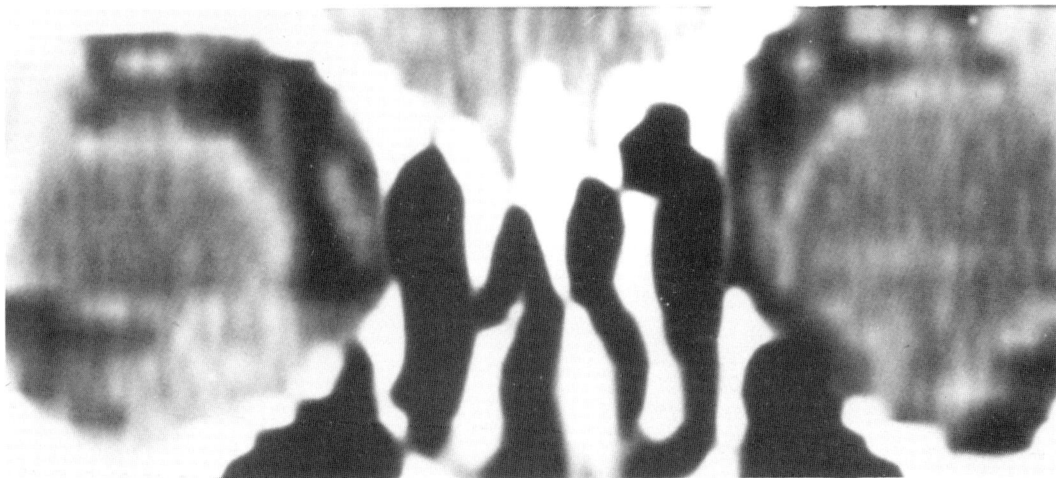

Figure 18C. Coronal reconstruction of Figure 18B.

2
Radiological Signs of Facial Injury

1. SUGGESTIVE SIGNS

A. Soft Tissue Swelling

Soft tissue swelling may decrease the transparency of a facial area after injury. On facial films, one may detect the hematoma produced at a contact point. The increased soft tissue density should signal the possibility of an underlying fracture.

Hematomas are most easily detected in the nasofrontal, periorbital, or malar areas on plain films (see Figure 21D).

CT examination has added a new aspect to facial injury by clearly depicting the soft tissues. Figure 19A illustrates the presence of periorbital and preseptal soft tissue swelling after injury. No fracture was found.

The patient depicted in Figure 19B had right proptosis and decreased vision following injury. In this axial view, the retrobulbar muscle cone was clear. Another view 6 mm higher shows a large hematoma (Figure 19C). An oblique lateral reconstruction in the plane of the globe and optic nerve, Figure 19D, shows the hematoma interposed between the orbital roof, upper muscle cone, and optic canal. No fracture was found.

B. Fluid in a Paranasal Sinus

Changes in transparency of a sinus should signal possible injury. An air-fluid level or complete opacity may, however, be the residual of antecedent sinus disease or simply indicate displacement of blood into a sinus secondary to a severe nosebleed.

Figure 20A is a plain radiograph in Waters position that shows an air-fluid (air-blood) level in the right maxillary sinus. Blood fills the left maxillary sinus so that it is completely opaque.

A similar air-fluid (air-blood) level is present in the axial CT of Figure 20B. On the right side, blood fills the posterior maxillary sinus, and a small

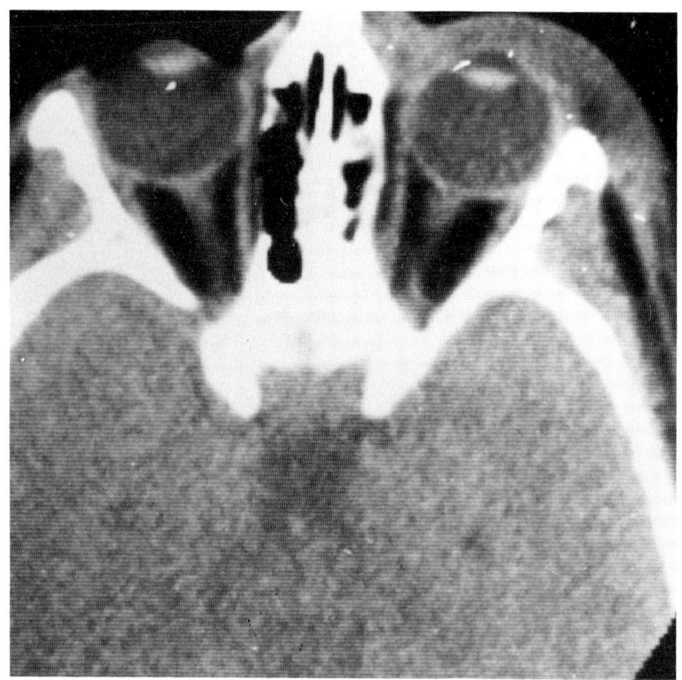

Figure 19A. CT in orbital soft tissue injury. Axial CT in midorbit plane from a patient with extensive preseptal periorbital hematoma on the right.

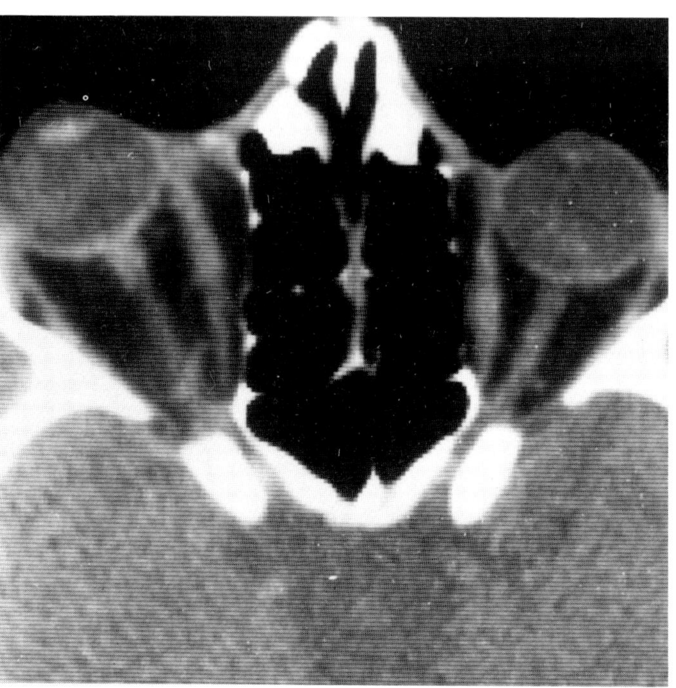

Figure 19B. Midorbit CT in patient with proptosis on right.

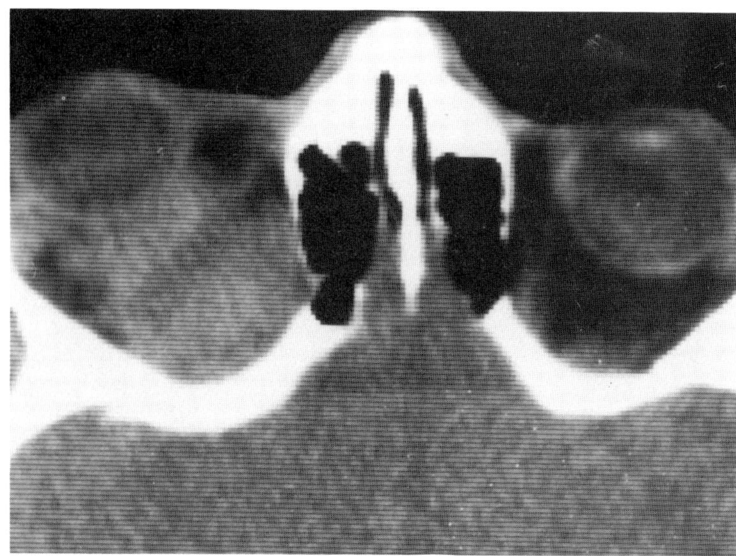

Figure 19C. Same patient, higher cut showing a large hematoma filling the posterior orbit.

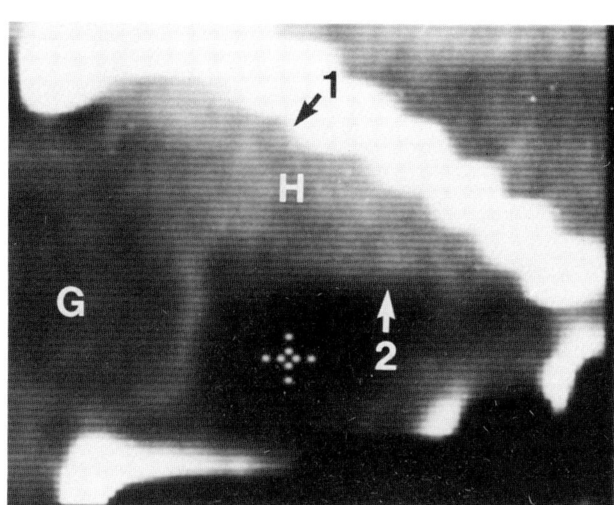

Figure 19D. Oblique reconstruction showing under orbital roof compressing globe, muscle cone, and optic nerve. G. Globe. H. Hematoma. 1. Orbital roof. 2. Inferior margin of optic nerve.

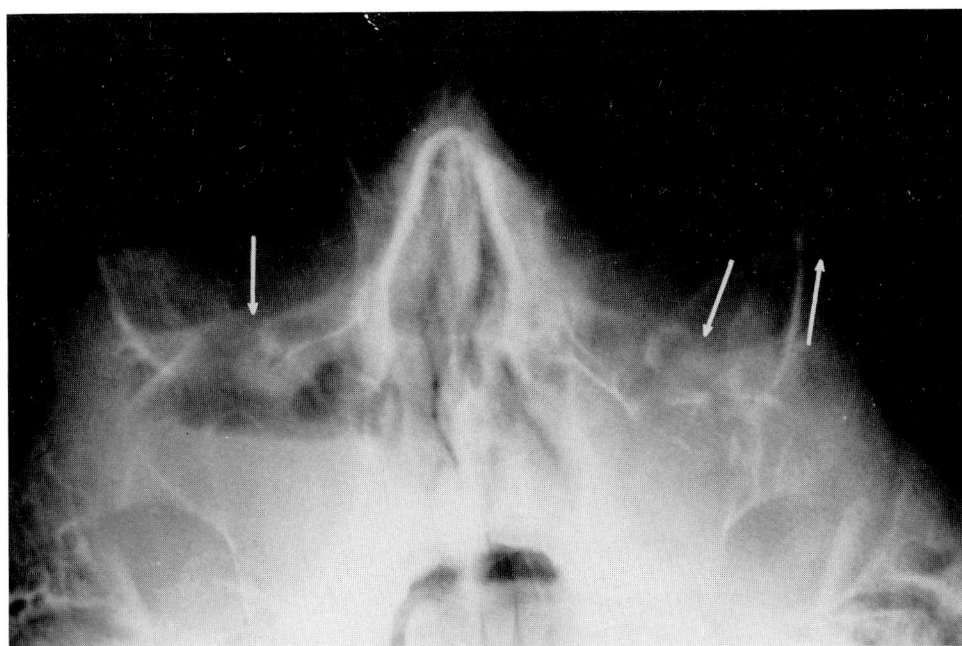

Figure 20A. Suggestive signs of injury and examples of the separation sign (cortical defect). Waters view patient with a LeFort II-left tripod fracture. Maxillary air-fluid level on the right side. Complete maxillary opacity is present on the left. Separation sign present in the inferior orbit rim on both sides and at the zygomaticofrontal suture on the left (arrows).

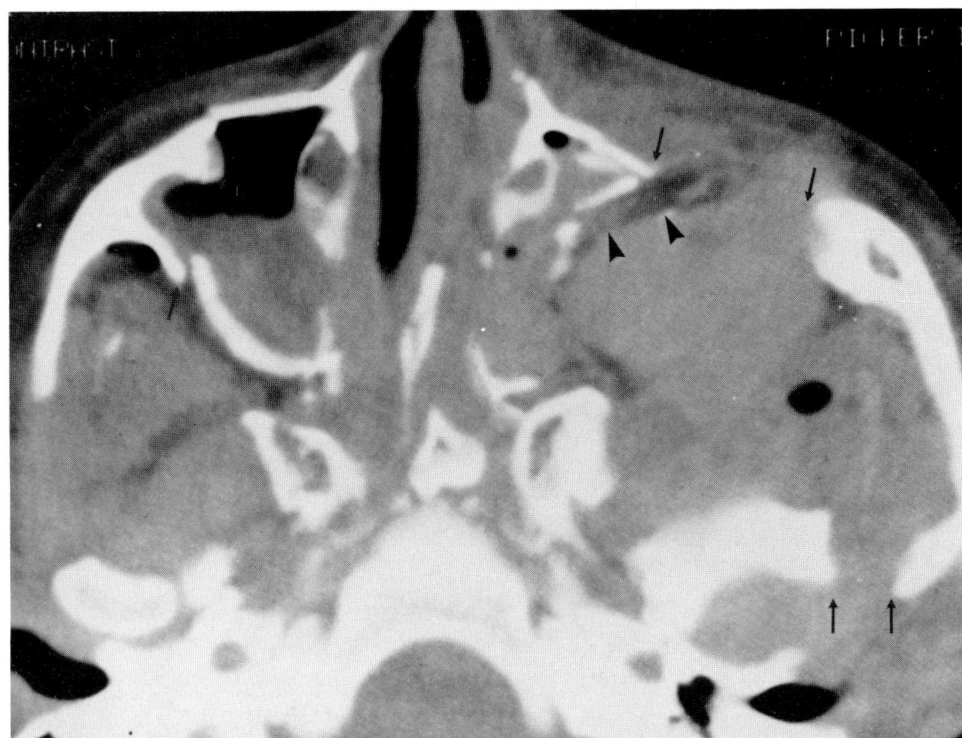

Figure 20B. CT slice from another patient with a LeFort II-left tripod injury more extensive than the previous injury. A right maxillary sinus air-fluid level is present while the left maxillary sinus is opaque. Retromaxillary fat is displaced against the crushed posterior maxillary sinus wall (arrowheads). Subtle separation of the right posterolateral maxillary sinus wall is present (single arrow). Gross anterior and posterior separation of the zygomatic arch is present on the left side (double arrows).

air accumulation is present anteriorly. In this case, the left maxillary sinus is completely interrupted, and rather complete opacity of the left side is present. Some retromaxillary fat can be seen adjacent to the compressed sinus lateral wall.

2. DIRECT SIGNS

When present, the following radiographic signs are consistant with facial injury. The principal difference in the radiographic appearance of each of these signs has to do with the way in which the bone fracture fragment is displaced in relation to surrounding bone.

A. Separation Sign (Cortical Defect)

If the fracture fragment is displaced away from surrounding bone, a small space is produced which on films produces an interruption in bone continuity.

Such an interruption is seen on the right side of the inferior orbital border in Figure 20A. A similar separation is present in the region of the left zygomaticofrontal suture and the left inferior orbital rim in this figure.

Subtle separation of the right lateral maxillary sinus wall is present in Figure 20B. Gross separation of the zygomatic arch from the maxillary attachment anteriorly and the temporal attachment posteriorly is present on the left side of this illustration.

B. Overlap Sign

If a compressive force produces a fracture, the fragment may be displaced so that it overlaps adjacent bone and produces a "double density" along the overlapping parts. Displacement of the anterior fragment of a zygomatic arch fracture in Figure 21A produces the overlap sign.

C. Abnormal Linear Density

When a fracture fragment is displaced so that it is turned in line with the long axis in the x-ray beam, a nonanatomical linear density area is produced. This sign has been termed the *abnormal linear density* by Merrell. Displacement of a lateral maxillary wall fragment produces the abnormal linear density in Figure 21B. Duplication of the OOL is due to the same sort of lateral orbital wall displacement.

D. "Disappearing" Fragment

This sign is the opposite of the abnormal linear density sign. A structure ordinarily producing a cortical absorption line in a normal patient may be

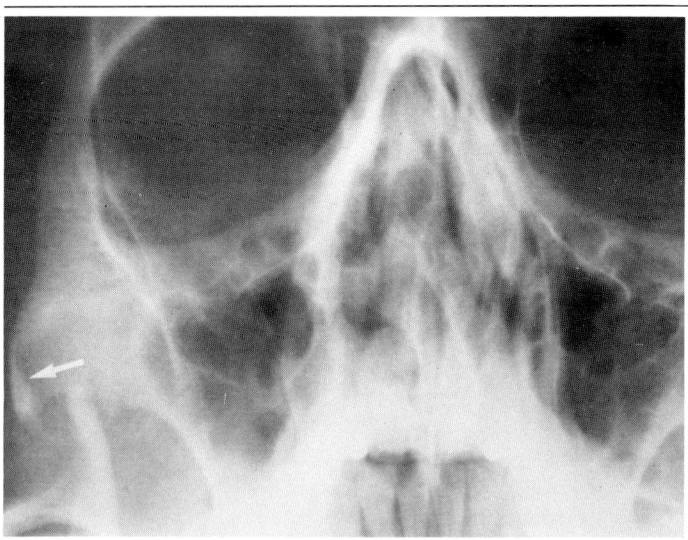

Figure 21A. Direct signs of fracture. Waters view of right zygomatic arch fracture with overlap sign at arrow.

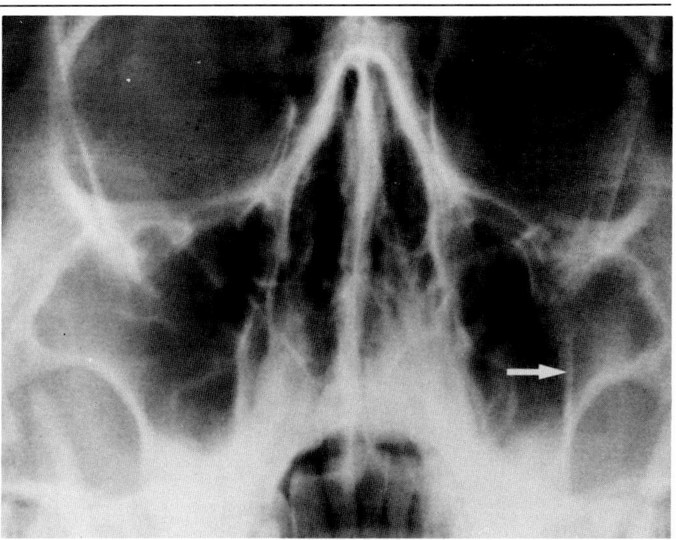

Figure 21B. Left tripod fracture with an abnormal linear-density area (arrow) due to a displaced maxillary wall fragment. Duplication of the left OOL due to displacement of a portion of the orbital process of the sphenoid.

rotated in position so that it seems to disappear after injury. In Figure 21C, a 2-cm palpable inferior orbital border fragment has been rotated out of the beam and seemingly has "disappeared." (As the reader may have assumed, the infraorbital nerve was injured and local numbness resulted after this injury.) After elevation, return to normal position, and fixation by metal sutures to adjacent stable bone, the rim appears normal as seen in Figure 21D.

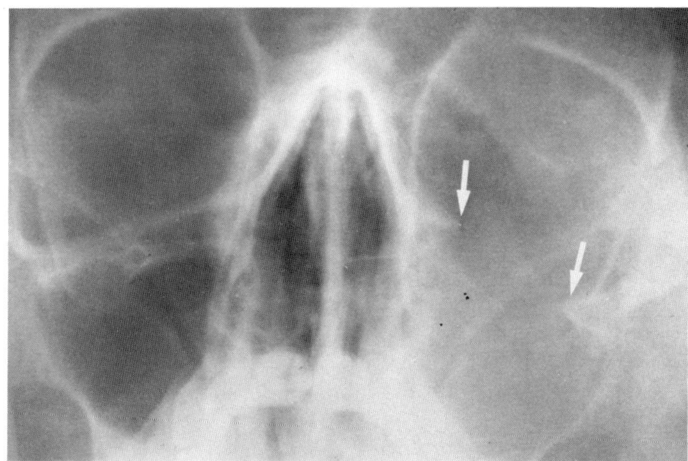

Figure 21C. Disappearing fragment of left inferior rim (arrows) after local fracture.

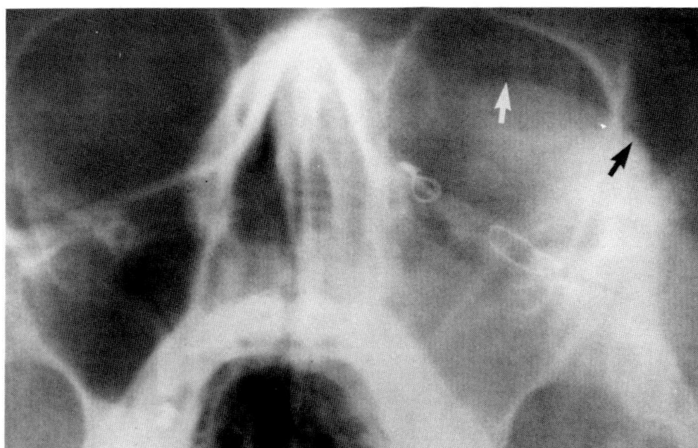

Figure 21D. Restoration and wire-suture fixation of fragment in Figure 21C. Arrows point to postoperative periorbital hematoma.

E. Periorbital or Subcutaneous Air

Periorbital air most commonly is the result of a lamina papyracea (ethmoidal) fracture. The nasal-frontal-ethmoidal complex injury in Figure 21E produced bilateral periorbital air (also see Figure 12).

We have also seen extensive facial subcutaneous air in patients with tripod fractures. This air escaped from the sinus when the patients blew their nose.

Intracranial air may result from a fracture through the posterior frontal sinus wall, ethmoidal roof, or sphenoidal sinus.

F. Displaced Structure

Injury may distort the position of a large fragment without revealing other definitive signs of a fracture on plain films. The patient depicted by Figure 21F has extensive displacement of the left nasal arch, frontal process of maxilla, and much of the inferior orbital rim. Structural displacement when compared to the opposite side is the main clue to this injury.

In other injury forms, there may be separation along one fracture margin and not others. This may occur frequently in the case of tripod fractures as described by Jacoby.

Fragment displacement is a frequent finding on CT examination of fractures.

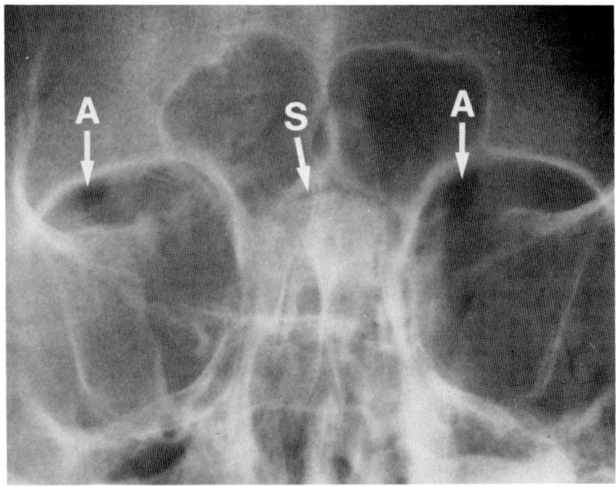

Figure 21E. Bilateral periorbital air (A, arrows). Nasal-frontal suture separation at S.

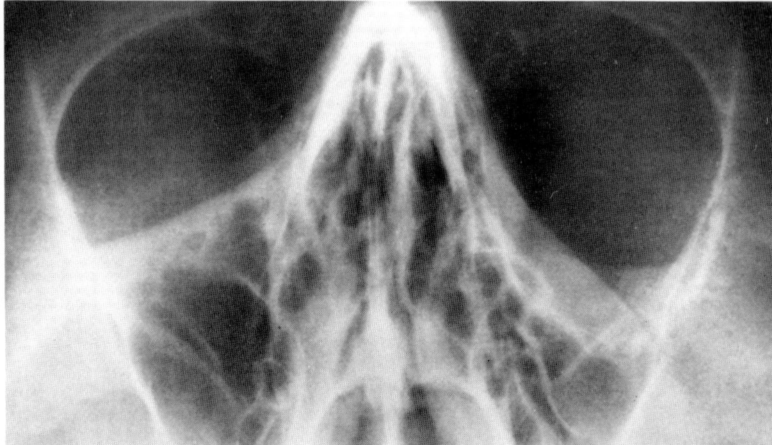

Figure 21F. Left nasal, frontal process of maxilla, and inferior orbital rim fragment displacement. Compare with opposite side.

3
Local Facial Injury

1. ORBIT FRACTURES

A portion of the orbit is involved in every other fracture form except the zygomatic arch fracture, local nasal fracture, and the LeFort I injury. Thus, evaluation of the orbital borders, orbital apex, and optic canal is a requisite part of any facial injury analysis.

Local injuries are considered in the following order:

Orbital floor (blowout) fracture

Lower orbital rim fracture

Nasal arch fracture

Zygomatic arch fracture

Upper orbital rim and frontal sinus fracture

A. Orbital Floor (Blowout) Fracture

By definition, the orbital blowout fracture excludes an interruption of the orbital rim. Compression of the ocular and periorbital soft tissues has been the typical mechanism of blowout fracture. In our experience, a blow by a fist is the most common cause of injury. Emery et al. report that more than half of the blowout fractures in their series were produced this way. We have also seen this injury as a result of a blow by an elbow, tennis ball, handball, or in auto accidents.

Diplopia and enophthalmos are considered the most common complications of a blowout fracture. Ocular injuries requiring treatment also occur and were present in 24% of the Emery series. Diplopia usually clears spontaneously. Enophthalmos may be present at the time of injury in the case of a large fracture fragment or may develop later as the periorbital hematoma is absorbed.

Hammerschlag's group was able to identify a blowout fracture, using the Waters and Caldwell views, in 97% of their cases. We agree that the majority of these fractures can be found on plain films.

The suggestive signs listed above are often present with a blowout fracture. Definitive bone spicules of a larger fragment should be the principal diagnostic criteria. The ethmoidal surface is involved in this fracture pattern in about 40% of cases.

Thin-section tomography plays an important part in blowout fracture evaluation. If surgery is considered, tomograms provide the best means of cross-section study of the orbital floor and lamina papyracea. CT may provide evidence of orbital floor disruption in axial or coronal section, but is a costly means of diagnosis. We reserve CT for study of complicated cases that cannot be resolved by more conventional study or when plain film examination fails to reveal a fracture that is clinically indicated by entrapment on the forced-duction test.

An undisplaced blowout fracture is illustrated by Figure 22A. Only a small soft tissue mass below the orbit floor is visualized on the Caldwell view in Figure 22B.

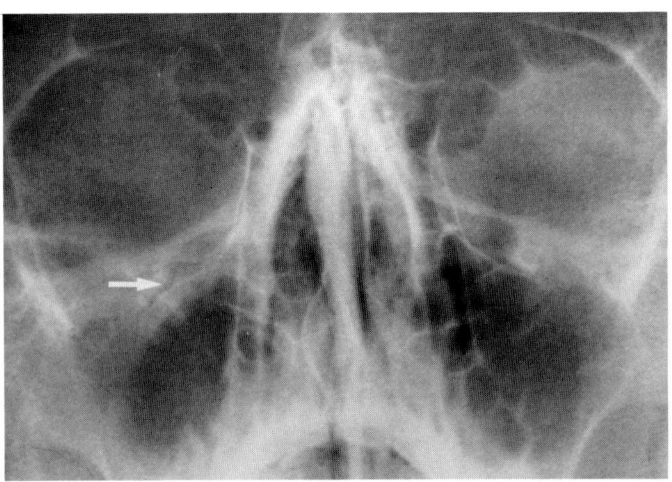

Figure 22A. Undisplaced right blowout fracture. Waters view with fracture line at arrow.

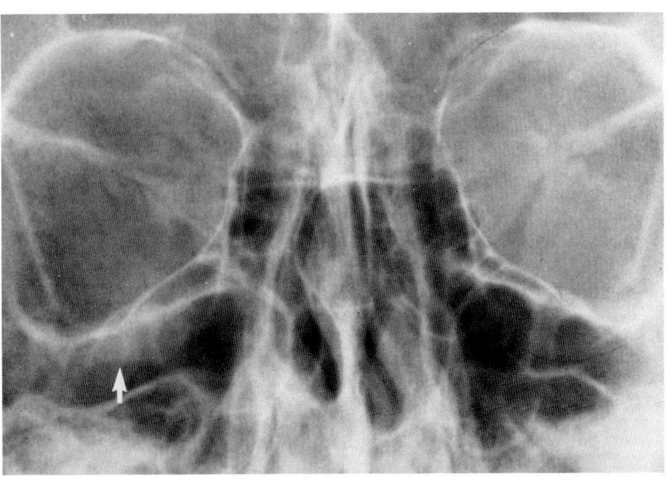

Figure 22B. Undisplaced right blowout fracture. Caldwell view shows only an oval mass in the right maxillary sinus at arrow.

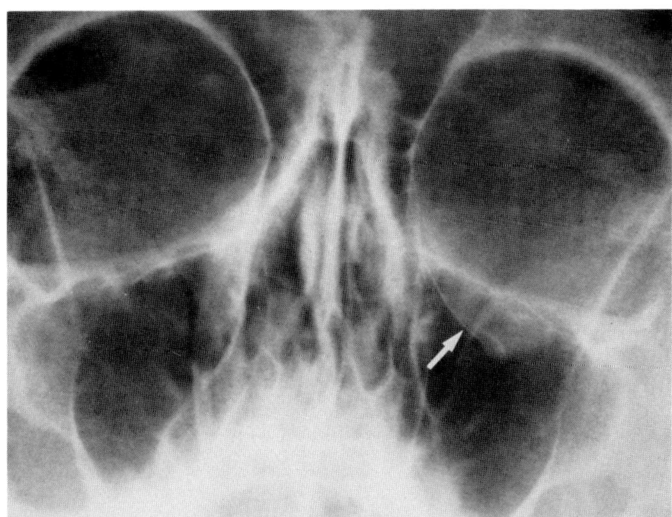

Figure 23A. Midfloor fracture on the left. Waters view. Arrow points to the fragment which simulates a trap door.

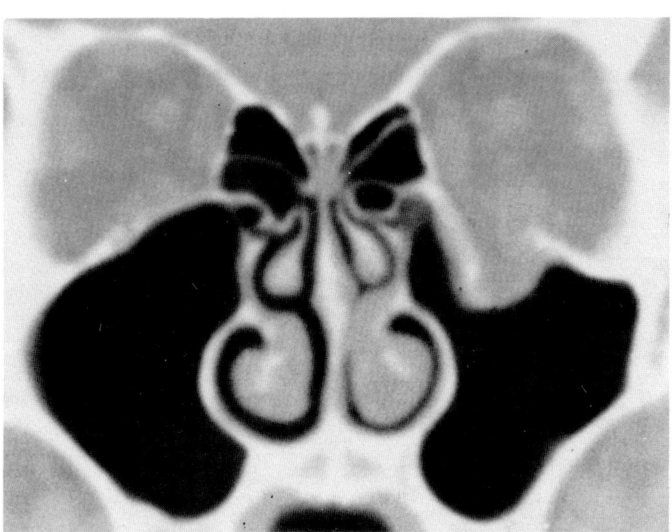

Figure 23B. Coronal CT examination reveals a "simple" orbital blowout fracture on the left.

Most often, the displaced blowout fracture fragment appears to be a trapdoor that is hinged toward the ethmoidal side of the orbit. This type of injury is demonstrated by Figure 23A. Periorbital fat produces the soft tissue density area protruding through the floor. Upward gaze was limited, and the forced-duction test was positive.

Coronal CT illustrates the "hinged" simple blowout fracture in Figure 23B. In this examination, the soft tissue periocular structures protrude through the orbit floor bone defect. The bone fragment seems to be hinged near the orbit floor—lamina papyracea junction medially. Wide separation of the orbit floor fracture edges is present laterally. Since the maxillary sinus mucoperiosteal lining tissue is intact, no blood is present in the sinus space. The lamina papyracea surface is intact.

While such CT examination is much more expensive than the plain radiographic studies, information about soft tissues of the orbit may aid the surgeon in evaluating the lesion. For example, in the soft tissue mode of this CT examination (not illustrated), the inferior rectus muscle lay above the soft tissues protruding into the maxillary sinus through the fracture. This encouraged the surgeon to follow the patient whose diplopia cleared in 2 weeks.

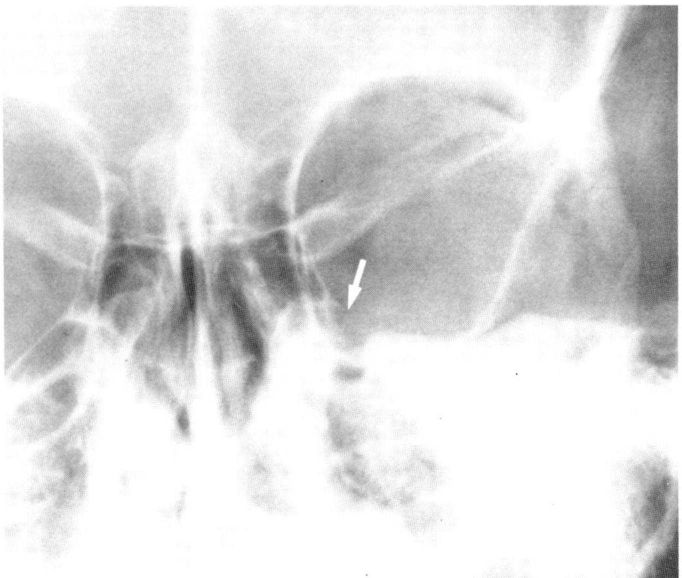

Figure 24A. Posterior blowout fracture on the left. The posterior floor cortex is absent on the left at arrow.

Figure 24B. An abnormal linear-density area at arrow represents the displaced floor in the Waters view.

Long-term follow-up revealed minimal enophthalmos, which was not noticeable cosmetically.

If the blowout displacement reaches the posterior orbital floor, the posterior cortical line seems to disappear (disappearing fragment sign) on the Caldwell view as seen in Figure 24A. Usually the displaced floor produces an abnormal linear density area as demonstrated in Figure 24B.

The use of tomography in an orbital floor and lamina papyracea blowout fracture is shown in Figure 25. The orbital volume enlargement produced

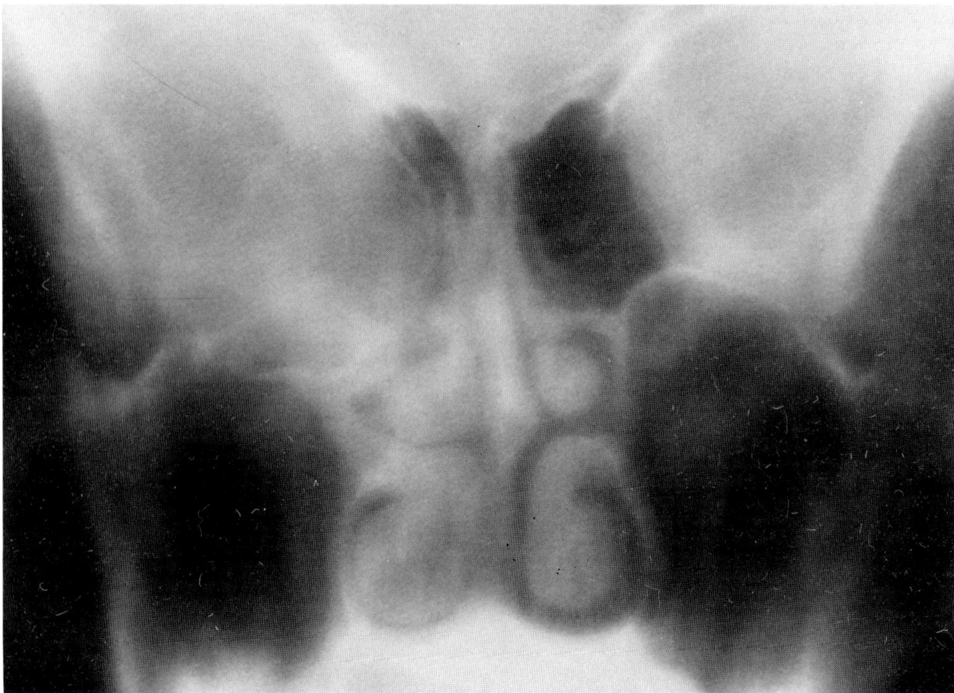

Figure 25. Marked medial displacement of the lamina papyracea and downward displacement of the right orbital floor in a tomographic study of a blowout fracture.

by this fracture easily explains the reason for persistent enophthalmos in this patient.

CT was helpful in delineating the very large defect produced by a left blowout fracture in the patient whose studies are shown in Figure 26. The Caldwell view, Figure 26A, demonstrates a large lamina papyracea and orbital floor defect. Deep enophthalmos is suggested by the broad, air-filled upper tarsal skin fold indicated by the arrows. Enophthalmos is confirmed by the midorbital axial CT examination in Figure 26B. This also shows a long ethmoidal surface indentation. The orbital floor and lower ethmoidal defect are confirmed in a lower axial CT, Figure 26C. The defects, especially that in the orbital floor are best seen in Figure 26D, the coronal CT.

CT examination may allow more complete evaluation of the large fragment orbital blowout fracture that is accompanied by a lamina papyracea fracture.

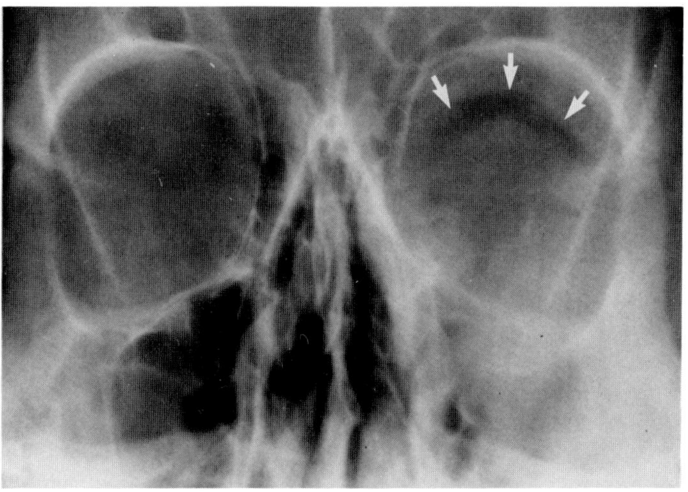

Figure 26A. Large left orbital floor and lamina papyracea defect. Caldwell view showing absent lamina and floor cortices. There is an opaque maxillary sinus. Prominent tarsal fold at arrows.

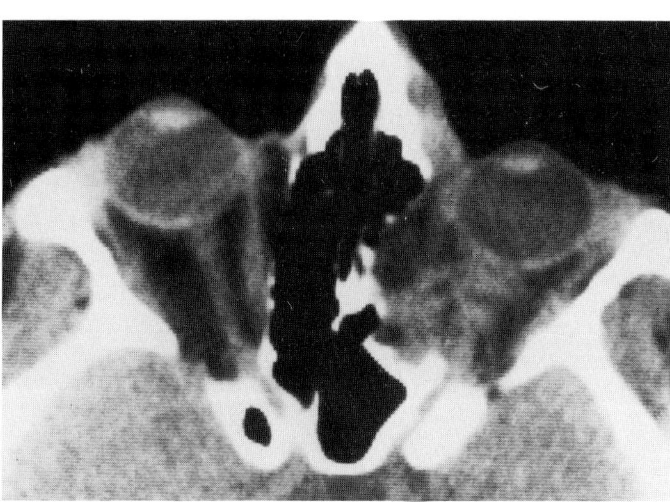

Figure 26B. Enophthalmos is present along with an ethmoidal surface defect in a midorbit axial CT.

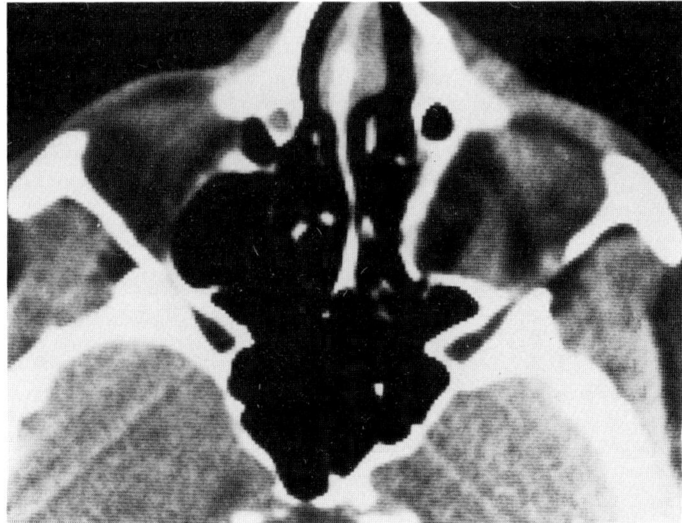

Figure 26C. The ethmoidal and orbital floor defects present in a low-axial orbital CT.

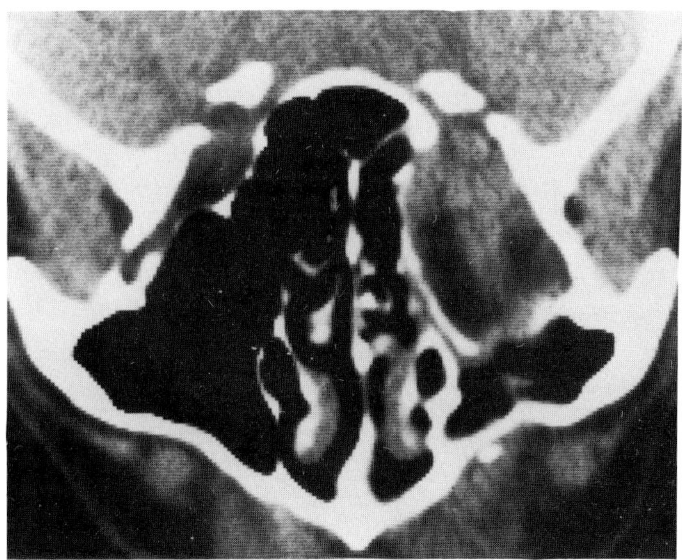

Figure 26D. Coronal CT shows the large defect.

This combination results in the greatest degree of orbital enlargement and thereby produces maximal enophthalmos. This type of injury most commonly requires early surgical restoration of orbital fragments to normal position. If surgery is delayed, later implantation of material to diminish the orbit size and to restore cosmetic symmetry may be necessary. Orbital implant application may also be required to reposition the ocular visual axis and overcome persistent diplopia.

The midmaxillary axial CT in Figure 27A shows displacement of the right orbit floor into the upper maxillary sinus, which produces sinus opacity on this side. Another view, Figure 27B made 6 mm higher, shows interruption and medial displacement of the entire lamina papyracea. The accompanying right ethmoidal sinus is also opacified by blood resulting from the injury.

An anterior coronal orbit CT, Figure 27C, in a plane immediately behind the globe confirms the orbit floor and lamina papyracea fractures by the ethmoid sinus opacity. It also shows the anterior portion of the orbit floor displacement and resulting enlargement in the size of the orbit when compared to the opposite side. A more posterior coronal CT, Figure 27D, demonstrates

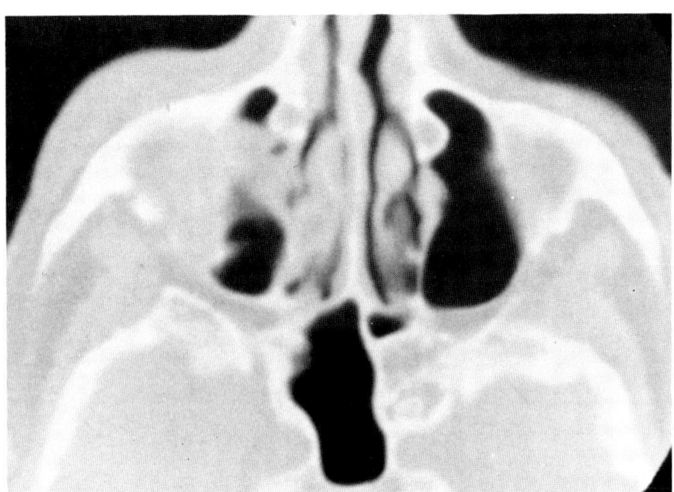

Figure 27A. CT of a large fragment blowout fracture. Axial CT demonstrates orbit floor displacement on the right.

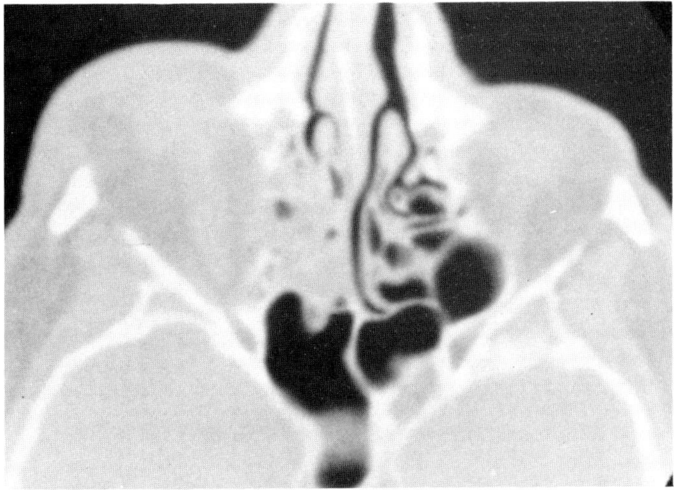

Figure 27B. Higher axial CT demonstrates fractures and displacement of the entire right lamina papyracea.

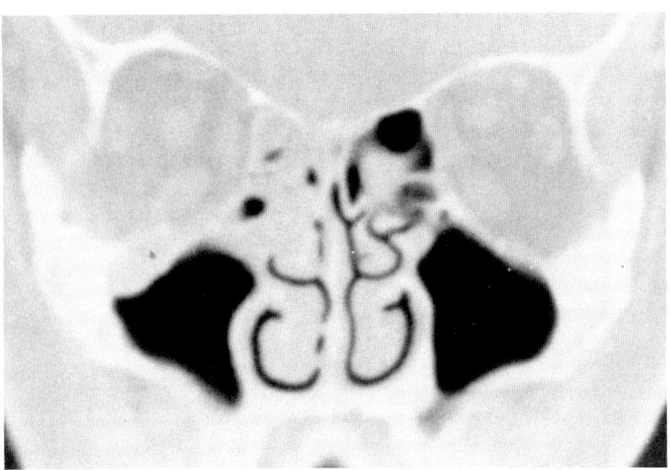

Figure 27C. An anterior coronal orbit CT confirms the orbit floor and lamina papyracea fractures.

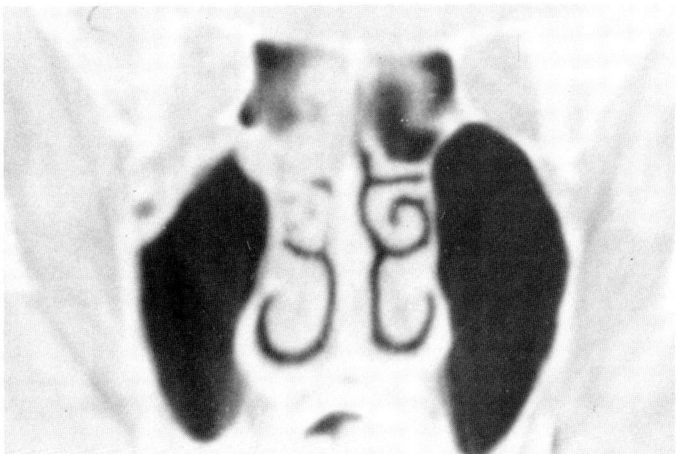

Figure 27D. A posterior coronal orbit CT demonstrates that the orbit floor fracture extends back to the inferior orbital fissure.

that the orbital floor fracture extends all the way back to the inferior orbital fissure. This floor fracture measured 24 mm in length. Information provided by this examination aided the surgeon in deciding on early restoration of the orbital floor position and thereby prevented enophthalmos and chronic diplopia.

B. Lower Orbital Rim Fracture

A blow directed to the lower orbital rim may produce a rim fragment such as that illustrated in Figures 21C and 21D. The direction of force produced a fragment rotation so that it seemed to disappear.

A more lateral segment of the inferior rim has been separated in the injury illustrated by Figure 28A. The fragment has been displaced downward and medially.

In many of the inferior orbital rim fractures, a portion of the anterior orbital floor is included in the fragment. Often the floor is obscured by the rim fragment. In Figure 28B, the left rim fracture (upper arrows) and displaced

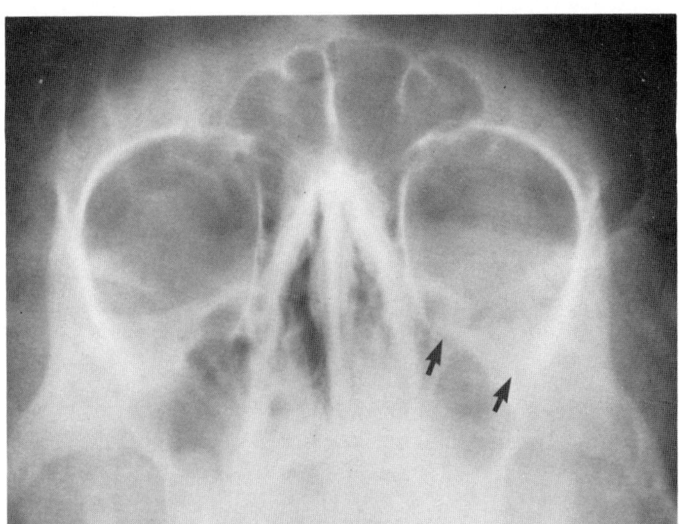

Figure 28A. Inferior orbital rim fracture. Downward and medial displacement of an outer rim fragment at arrows.

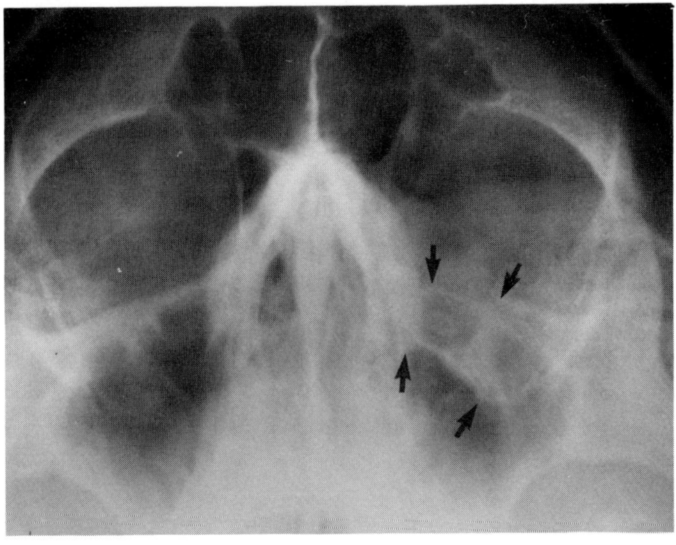

Figure 28B. Orbital rim fracture at upper arrows. Orbital floor fragment at lower arrows.

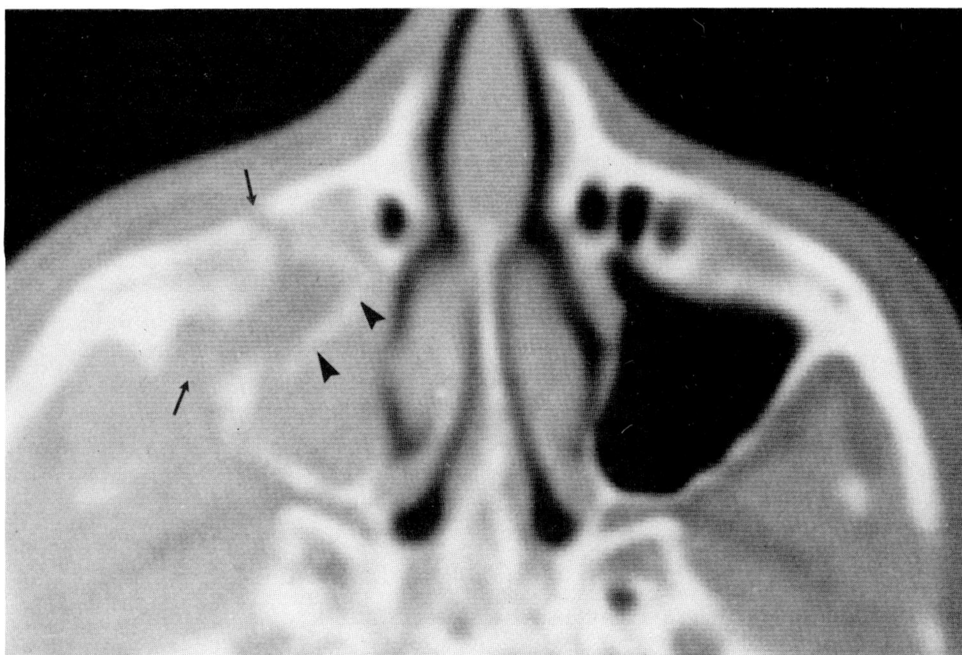

Figure 28C. An axial CT view shows a fracture through the inferior orbit rim that extends obliquely across the zygomaticomaxillary suture area (arrows). A portion of the orbit floor is displaced into the opaque maxillary sinus (arrowheads).

orbital floor (lower arrows) are both evident. Less apparent is the lamina papyracea fracture indicated by a thickening along the medial surface of the orbit.

Axial CT of the lower orbital rim fracture usually demonstrates the accompanying orbit floor involvement as well. Figure 28C reflects this change. The lower rim is interrupted, an oblique fracture extends along the maxillary-zygoma suture plane, and a portion of the orbit floor is rotated into the opaque maxillary sinus.

C. Nasal Arch Fracture

Nasal tip fractures are commonplace isolated injuries best visualized on the underexposed lateral view. This view also can be used to define more severe injury to the bony margins of the nasal fossa. Interruption of the anterior nasal spine and premaxilla may also be defined by the lateral view.

The patient illustrated by Figure 29A has extensive injury of the maxillary margins of the nose, anterior nasal spine, and premaxilla. All of these fractures have their fragment separation oriented to the transverse plane. While an injury of the nasal arch might be suspected from the changes on the lateral view in Figure 29A, no direct evidence of such injury is present on the lateral view.

Since the nasal arch is oriented in a longitudinal plane, it is best seen in the Waters view. Figure 29B is from the same examination as Figure 29A. In the Waters view, both nasal bones have been separated from the perpendicular plate of the ethmoid and from both maxillary frontal processes. The left

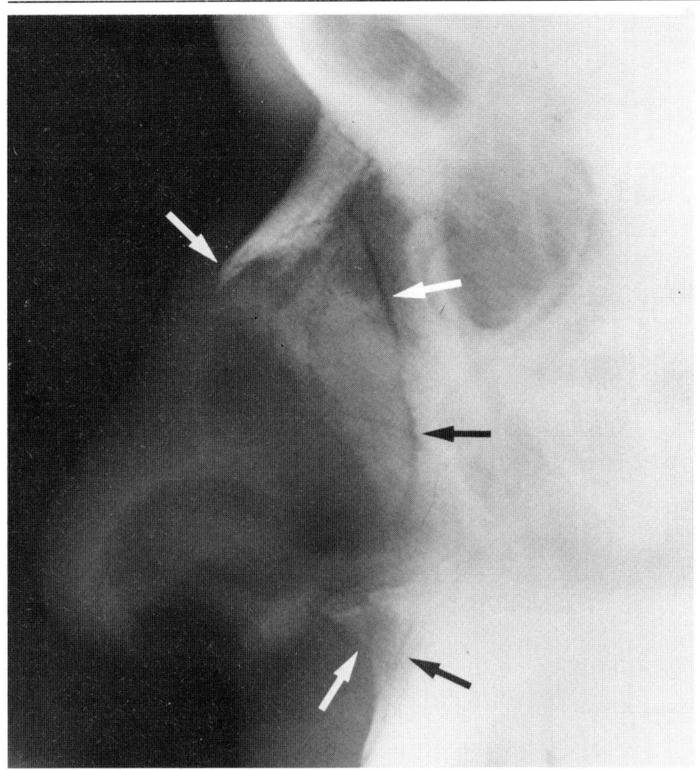

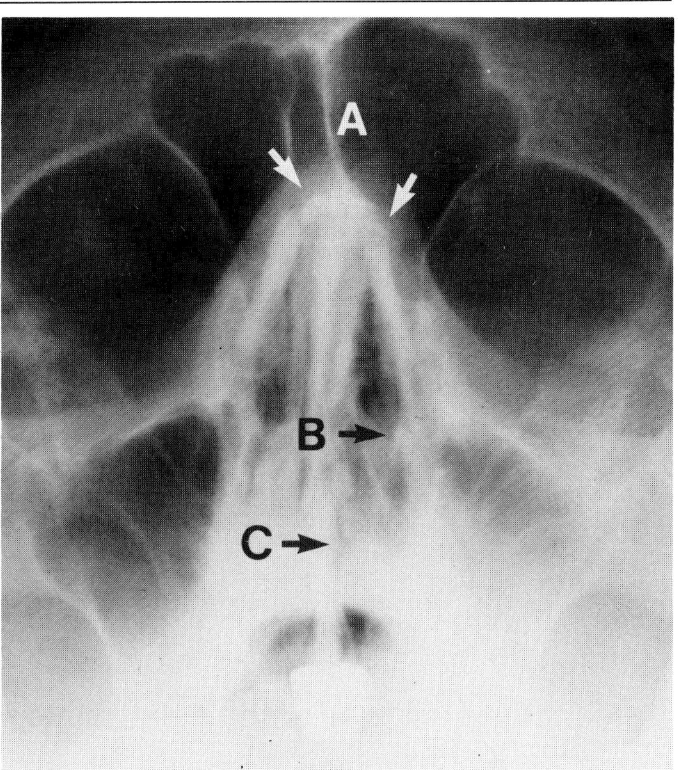

Figure 29A. Extensive nasal injury. Lateral view with nasal tip fracture at upper arrow, frontal process of maxilla at middle arrows, and anterior nasal spine fracture at lower arrows.

Figure 29B. Waters view shows a nasal arch fracture at A, frontal process fracture at B, and a portion of the premaxilla fracture at C.

frontal process has been interrupted along the medial border of the maxillary sinus producing the sinus opacity. A portion of the premaxilla injury can be seen between the central incisors.

The facial surgeon is concerned about the airway and cosmetic appearence of the patient with a nasal injury. Therefore, information such as that gained about the last patient can be very helpful to the surgeon.

Nasal arch interruption may also signal more extensive injury of the orbital rim, orbital floor, ethmoidal sinus, and frontal sinus.

The left nasal bone and frontal process are separated from the remaining arch in Figure 30A. The frontal process is separated also along the medial maxillary sinus border and at the medial edge of a displaced orbital rim fragment. The nasal bone and frontal process form a large fragment that has the shape of an inverted Y at the arrows. The entire orbital floor has been displaced downward. An accompanying Caldwell view, Figure 30B, shows the associated left lamina papyracea fracture and further demonstrates the extent of the orbital floor fracture.

While the interruption of the frontal process of the maxilla can easily be demonstrated on plain films, CT is necessary to show the accompanying separation of the adjacent lacrimal canal from the lamina papyracea. Figure 30C illustrates posterior displacement of the frontal process of the maxilla accompanied by a lamina papyracea fracture, which isolates the structures about the lacrimal bony canal. Lateral displacement of this complex is also present.

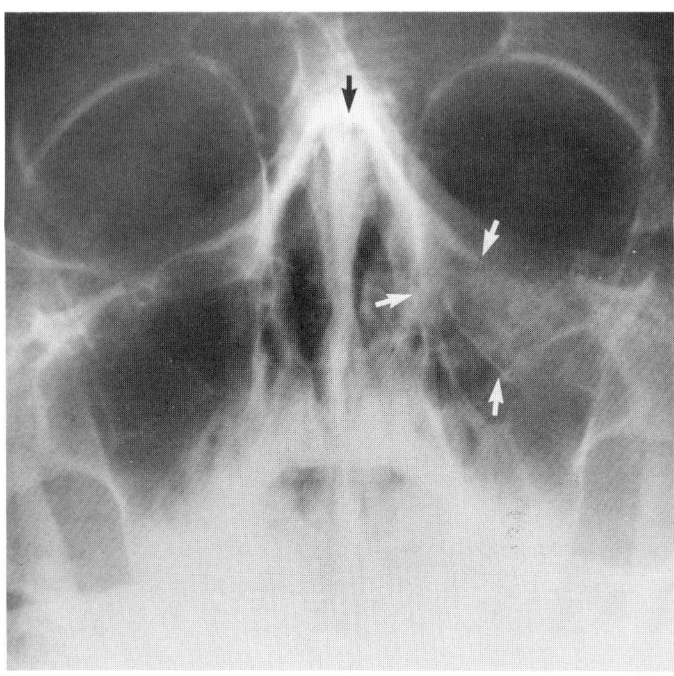

Figure 30A. Left nasal arch fracture with frontal process, orbital rim, and floor involvement. Inverted Y of left nasal bone and frontal process of maxilla at upper arrows. Orbital rim "disappearing fragment." Orbital floor fracture at lower vertical arrow.

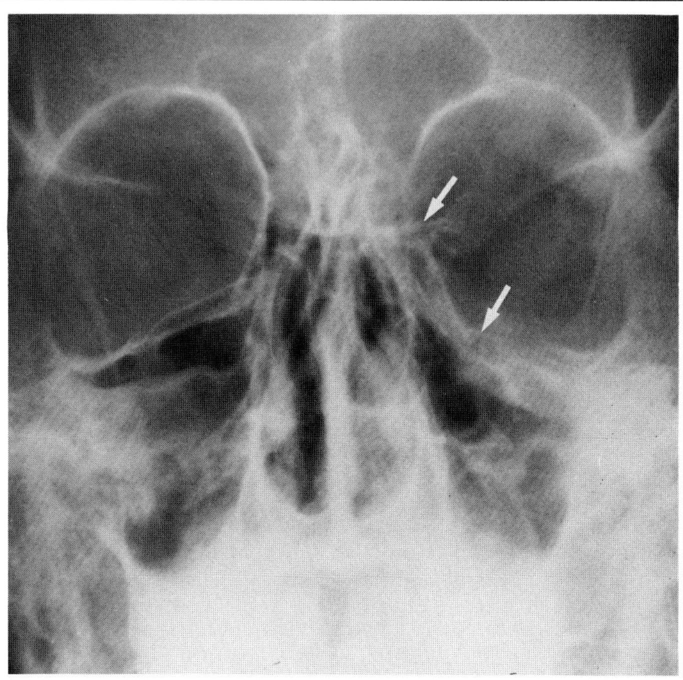

Figure 30B. Lamina papyracea fracture at arrows.

Lacrimal duct membranous injury with epiphora usually accompanies such a frontal process–lacrimal bony canal injury.

Quite often medial orbital soft tissue injury accompanies the lamina papyracea fracture component underlying the frontal process–lacrimal bony canal complex injury. As seen in Figure 30D, a sizable hematoma is present alongside the lamina papyracea fracture. The hematoma extends to the supra-orbital vein region and on other cuts displaced the attachment of the superior oblique ocular muscle. The lamina papyracea fracture may also extend su-

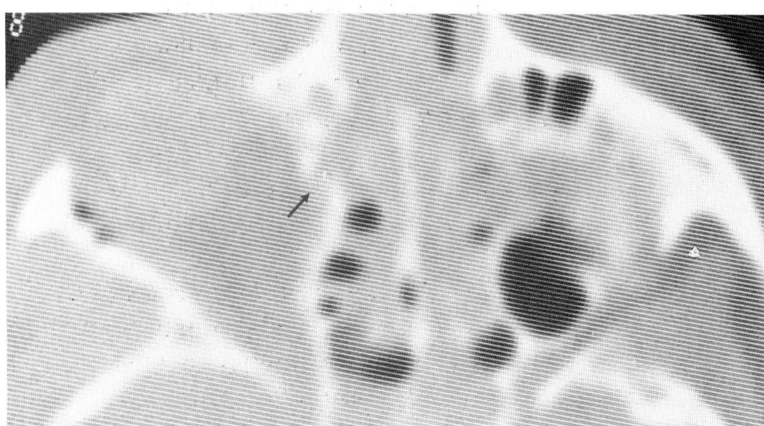

Figure 30C. A midorbital axial CT shows a lamina papyracea fracture that separates the frontal process–lacrimal bony canal complex (arrow). Posterior and lateral displacement of the complex is present.

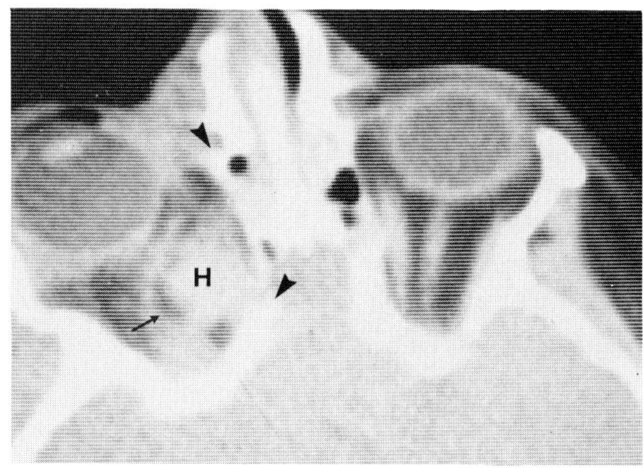

Figure 30D. An axial CT 12 mm higher shows a large lamina papyracea fragment (arrowheads) with a hematoma (H) that extends to the superior ophthalmic view (arrow).

periorly, as it did in this patient, to involve the ethmoid roof—cribriform plate area and produce cerebrospinal fluid rhinorrhea. Hematoma and infection can also affect the anterior cranial fossa through this ethmoidal route.

A force applied to the left frontal, nasal, and orbital area produced the injury depicted by Figure 31. A stellate frontal sinus fracture extends along and interrupts the upper inner border of the left orbital margin in Figure 31A. The nasal arch is comminuted and displaced downward. The perpendicular plate and vomer are separated in the center of the nasal septum. Rotation of the frontal process and inferior orbital rim fragment have resulted in a step-like deformity of the inferior rim, and the orbital floor is interrupted. In the Caldwell view, Figure 31B, the left frontal process displacement can be seen, and a blood clot opacifies the frontal sinus. Figure 31C is a lateral view that

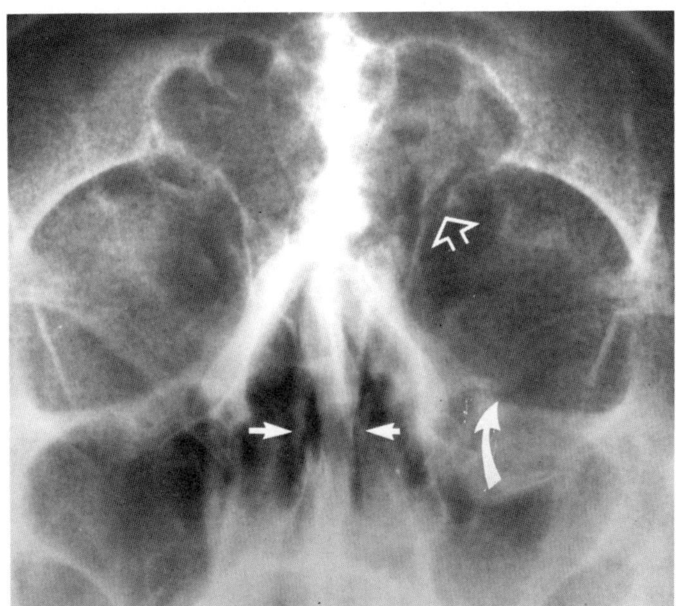

Figure 31A. Frontal sinus stellate fracture with depressed nasal arch, septum fracture, frontal process displacement, and orbital floor fracture. Waters view with stellate frontal fracture and upper orbital rim fracture at upper vertical arrow. Rotated frontal process step-off with lower rim at lower vertical arrow. Septum fracture at horizontal arrows.

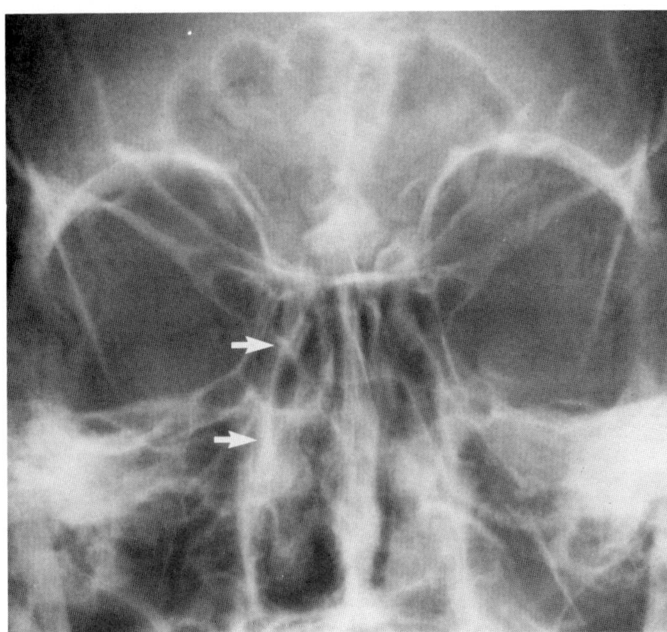

Figure 31B. Left frontal process displacement—compare with normal right at arrows. Opaque frontal sinus.

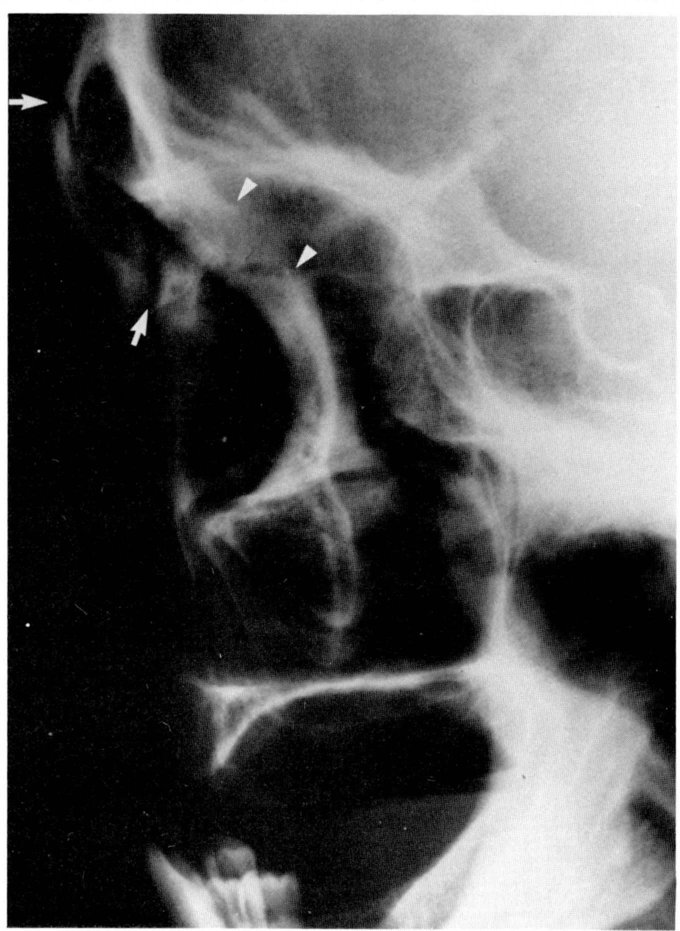

Figure 31C. Lateral view with frontal fracture margins at white arrows and ethmoidal roof separation at arrowheads.

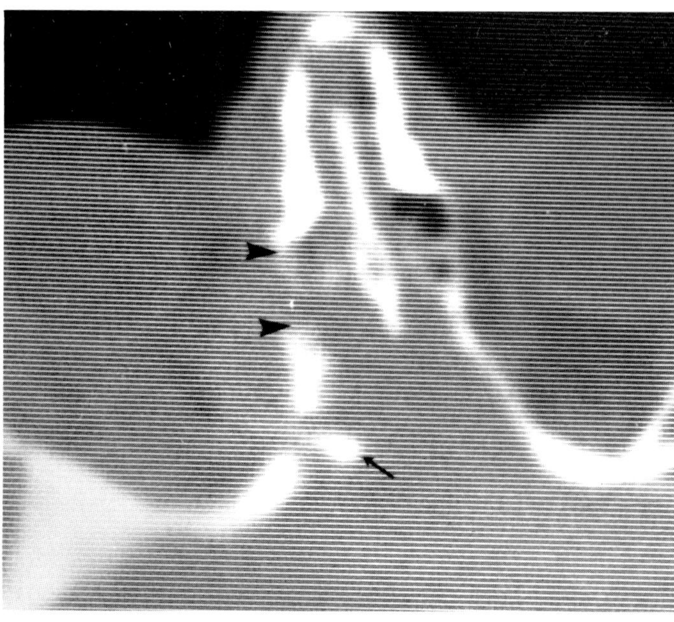

Figure 31D. An axial upper orbit CT shows several fractures (arrowheads) of the orbit roof border. One rotated fragment (arrow) present. Subtle nasal longitudinal fractures present.

shows the upper and lower margins of the frontal sinus fracture, as well as ethmoidal roof fractures. These changes should suggest that the patient may develop a cerebrospinal fluid leak.

These cases illustrate how extensive central axis and orbital injury may accompany an interruption of the nasal arch.

Nasal arch fractures may be very subtle in CT examination due to the oblique position of the nasal bones. Longitudinal nasal fractures were present in the patient whose injury is illustrated in Figure 31D. These fractures are overshadowed by the medial and lateral orbital roof fractures. One fragment along the medial border of the orbit represents a piece of bone originally oriented in an anteroposterior position, but rotated 90° by the compressive force on the upper orbit so that it lies in a horizontal position.

On a slightly higher view in Figure 31E, upward continuation of the fractures into the orbital roof can be seen. Such injury of the orbit roof should signal the possibility of accompanying anterior fossa or frontal lobe brain injury.

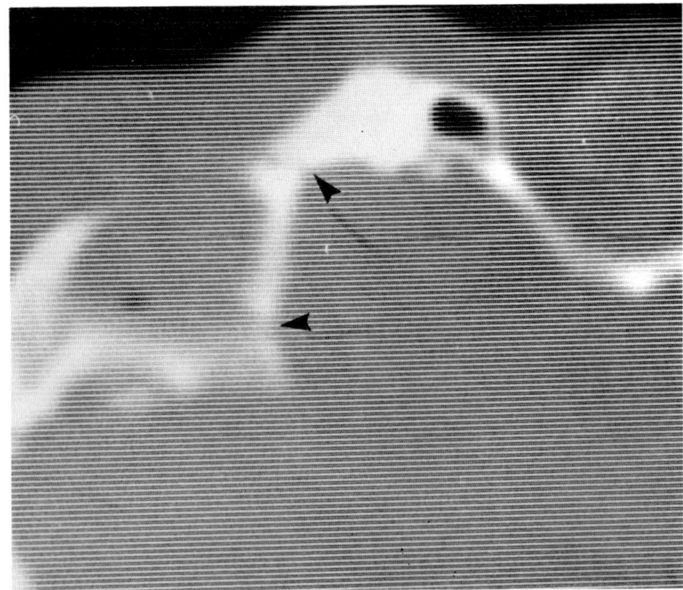

Figure 31E. A slightly higher axial CT shows the orbit roof continuity of these fractures (arrowheads).

D. Zygomatic Arch Fracture

The zygomatic arch is vulnerable to a blow from the lateral direction that produces a central inbending fracture and accompanying outbending fractures in the zygomatic and temporal portions of the arch. This position is easily detected in the Waters projection as seen in Figure 21A.

Occasionally, the anterior outbending portion of a zygomatic arch fracture may involve the zygoma body and orbital process. The Waters view in Figure 32A demonstrates an indentation of the zygomatic arch and temporal outbending typical of the arch fracture. More anteriorly, the other outbending fracture is through the orbital process and body of the zygoma. The latter change is especially evident in Figure 32B, the Caldwell view.

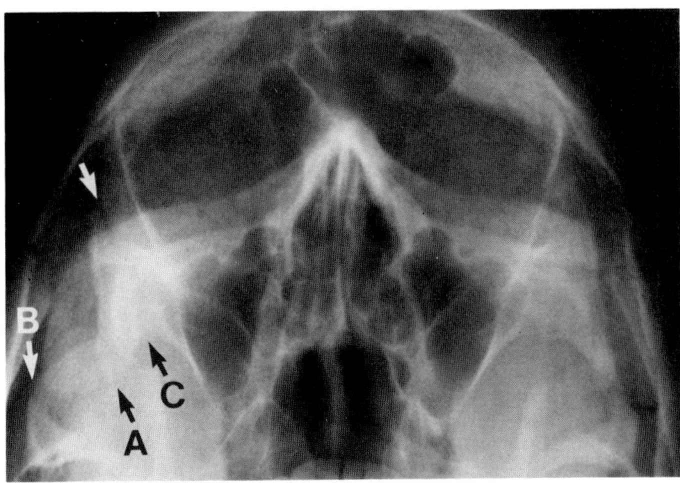

Figure 32A. Zygomatic arch fracture with anterior component through the zygoma body and orbital process. Waters view. In-bending at A. Temporal process outbending at B. Perpendicular outbending through zygoma at C.

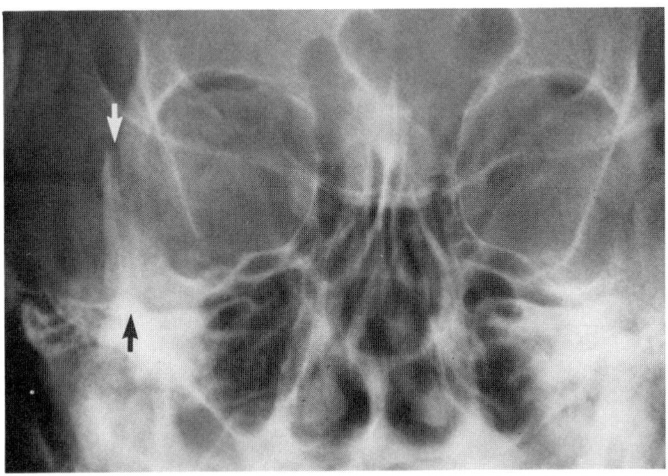

Figure 32B. A Caldwell view shows extension of the fracture along the outer portion of the orbital process (arrows).

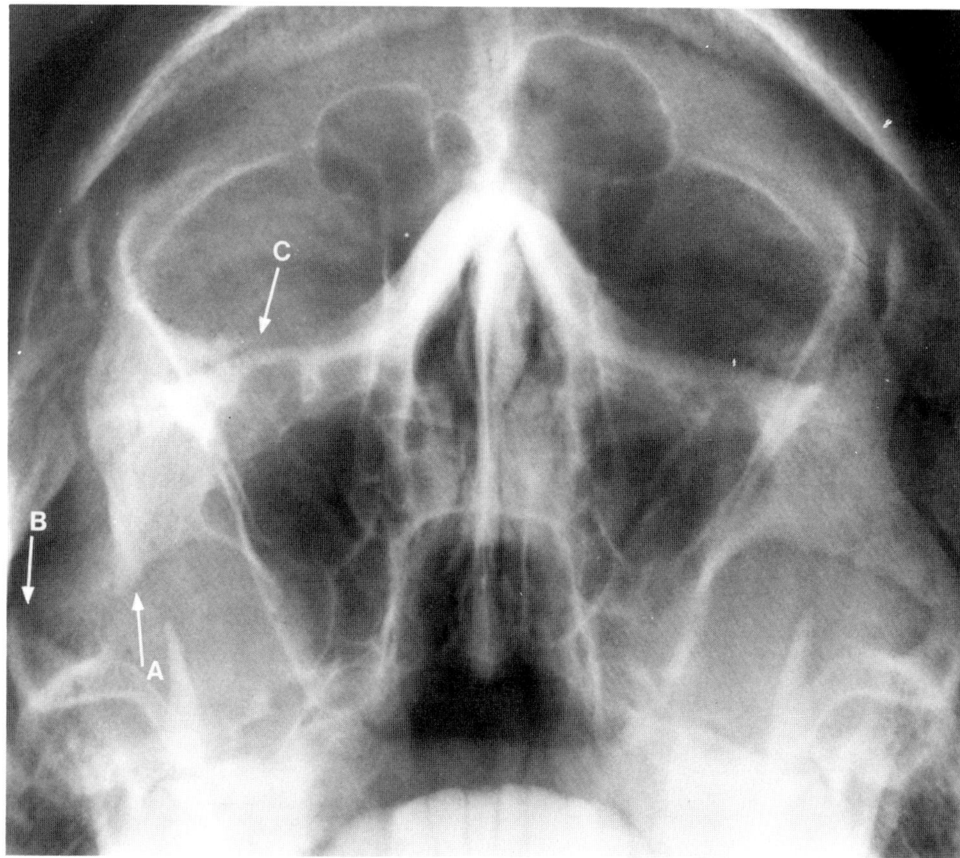

Figure 33. Zygomatic arch fracture with transverse extension of the anterior fracture through the zygoma body. Inbending of arch at A. Temporal process outbending at B. Transverse zygoma fracture at C.

Rarely the zygomatic arch fracture will be accompanied by a transverse fracture through the zygoma body as seen in Figure 33.

E. Upper Orbital Rim and Frontal Sinus

The upper orbital rim is infrequently fractured, but may become especially vulnerable if the frontal sinus is large in size as seen in Figure 34. Two large upper orbital rim fragments have been displaced downward as seen in Figure 34A. Tomograms demonstrated only involvement of the anterior upper rim and outer sinus wall.

Following reduction, the outer fragment was wired to the stable orbital process of the frontal bone. The medial fragment was then anchored to the stabilized outer fragment by another wire suture. Comminution prevented suturing of the medial fracture, but as seen in Figure 34B, the upper inner orbit was held in good position by soft tissues.

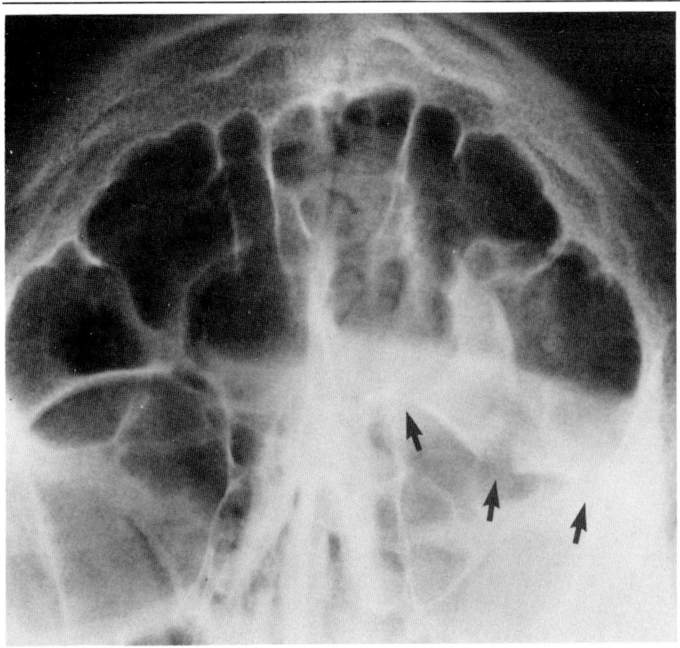

Figure 34A. Upper orbital rim fracture in a patient with a large frontal sinus. Fractures at arrows produce two large fragments that are displaced downward.

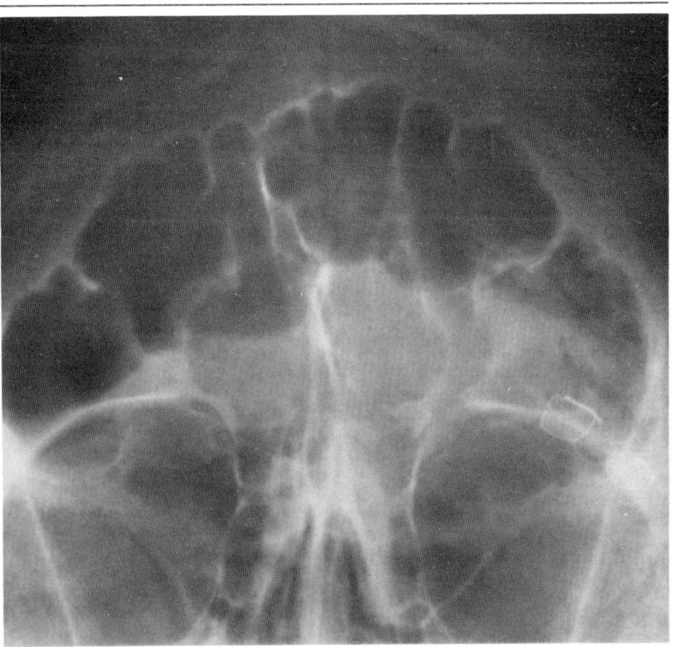

Figure 34B. Following reduction and fixation the upper orbital border has been replaced in position.

More extensive force application results in orbital roof, ethmoidal, and orbital floor fractures as seen in Figure 35. In this patient, the entire right upper orbital rim and adjacent frontal sinus is comminuted, the lamina papyracea is also fractured, and a long-segment orbit floor fracture is present. One would expect a detachment of the trochlear sling for the superior oblique muscle and a cerebrospinal fluid leak would probably develop. The patient's vision was intact.

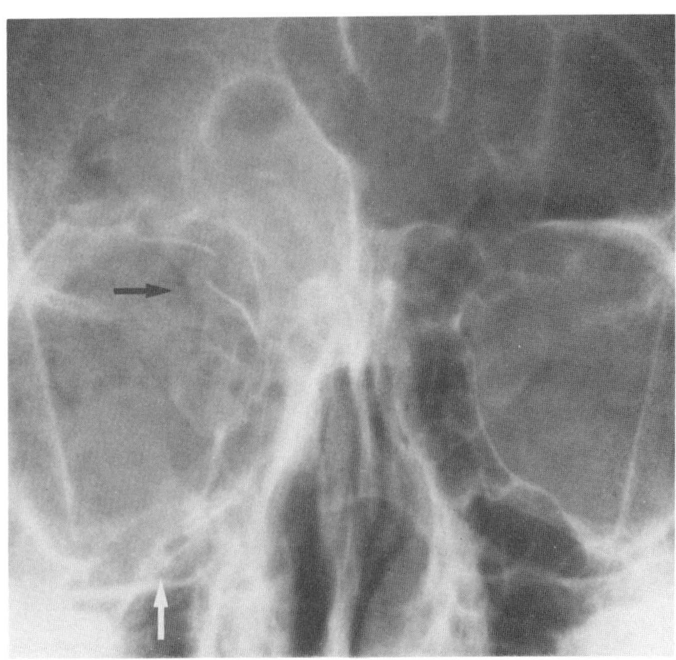

Figure 35. Comminuted fracture involving the right upper orbital rim, the frontal sinus, and ethmoidal sinus. A longitudinal orbital roof fracture (upper arrow) extends posteriorly through the lesser wing. A blowout fracture is present at the lower arrow.

CT may be very helpful in the study of fractures involving the frontal sinus, but does not demonstrate the upper orbital rim to good advantage. The frontal sinus anterior surface fracture is well defined in Figure 36A. Lower CT views failed to show comminuted fragments along the upper inner orbital rim, whereas these were quite evident on plain films. One might also be misled into thinking a large fracture fragment is present by the appearance of the normal superior orbital neurovascular grooves as seen in Figure 36B.

A coronal CT view of this patient is illustrated by Figure 36C. The marked enlargement of the right orbit is better defined than on plain examination. The upper, outer, medial, and inferior orbit borders are all fractured and displaced to produce an orbital "bursting" injury. The fracture through the frontal sinus was found on other more anterior views (not illustrated).

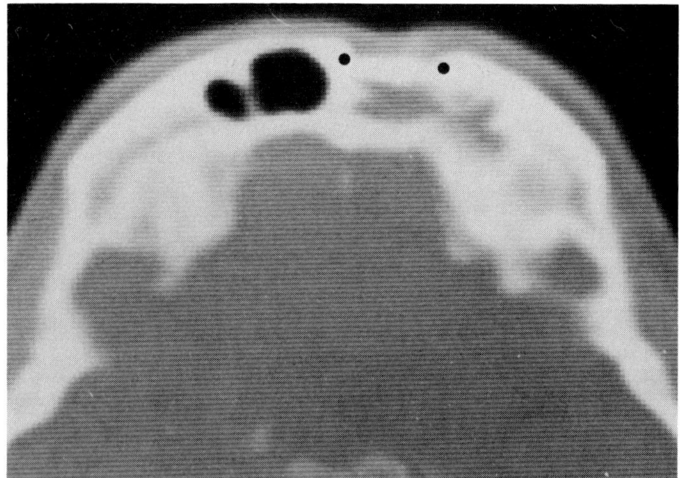

Figure 36A. Comminuted, depressed left frontal sinus anterior wall and inner upper orbital rim fracture. Upper CT with depressed anterior frontal sinus wall.

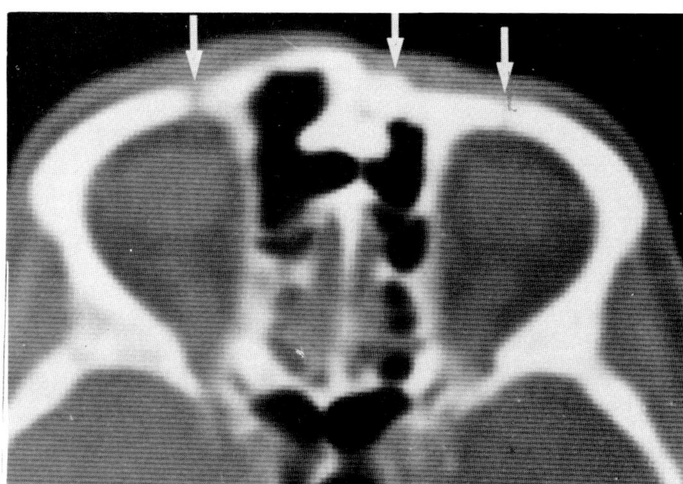

Figure 36B. Lower level with fracture at central arrow. Outer arrows indicate normal supraorbital neurovascular grooves.

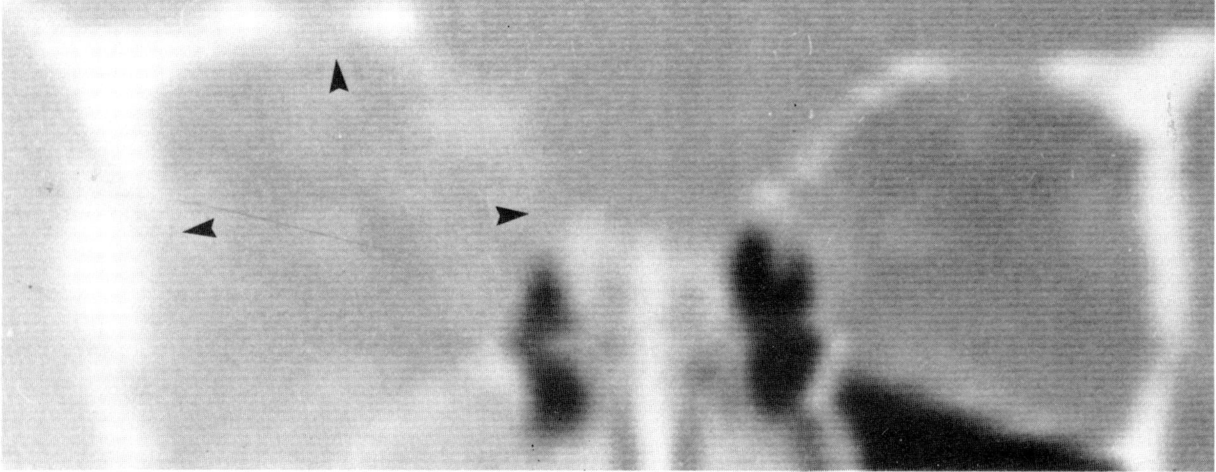

Figure 36C. Coronal CT reconstruction of an orbit "burst" fracture. Fractures of each margin of the orbit (arrowheads) have resulted in an enlarged orbit on the right.

4

The Tripod Fracture and Frontal Process Fracture

1. THE TRIPOD FRACTURE

A number of regional terms have been applied to the fracture form involving the attachments of the zygoma, including *the zygomaticomaxillary complex, zygomaticofacial*, trimalar, and tripod fractures.

We prefer, and use, the term *tripod fracture*, because this best reflects the "three-legged stool" arrangement of the zygoma and its principal attachments. A narrow, posteriorly directed temporal process helps form the zygomatic arch. Superiorly, the zygomatic orbital process unites with the orbital process of the frontal bone at the sygomaticofrontal suture. The orbital process also has a thin posterior lamella that unites with the orbital process of the sphenoid to form the lateral orbital wall. The broadest and most supportive part of the zygoma is the maxillary process, which covers the superolateral margin of the maxillary sinus and, in the well-developed sinus, is pneumatized by the zygomatic recess of the sinus. The orbital portion of the zygomaticomaxillary suture nearly reaches the infraorbital foramen.

The tripod fracture results in separation of the zygoma from the three major bone attachments; hence, the tripod fracture implies an interruption of all three legs.

An example of a left tripod fracture is illustrated in Figure 37. Force application was over the zygoma body in a medial and posterior direction. An air-fluid level is present in the maxillary sinus, and an oblique fracture line spans the outer maxilla. Elevation of the movable outer orbital border is present. The lateral maxillary mobile portion is displaced medially. A separation line is present in the zygomatic arch. All of these features are evident in Figure 37A, the Waters view.

The Caldwell view best shows the zygomaticofrontal suture separation as demonstrated in Figure 37B. The lateral orbital wall fracture is not evident.

The right tripod fracture fragment in Figure 38A has been displaced downward so that the outer (mobile) orbital rim fragment lies below the level of the stable medial orbital rim. The lateral maxillary portion of the fracture has been displaced medially producing a double line just above the alveolus.

"

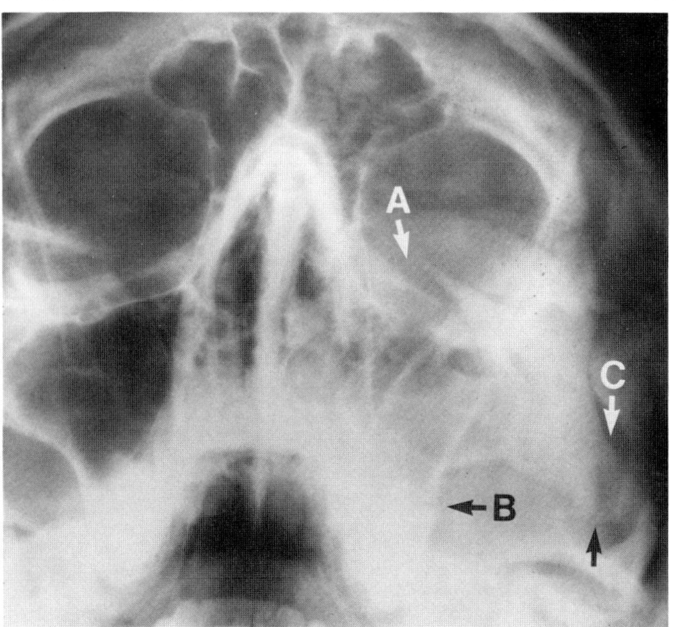

Figure 37A. A left tripod fracture. Waters view with orbital rim interruption at A. Lateral maxillary fracture at B. Undisplaced zygomatic arch fracture at C.

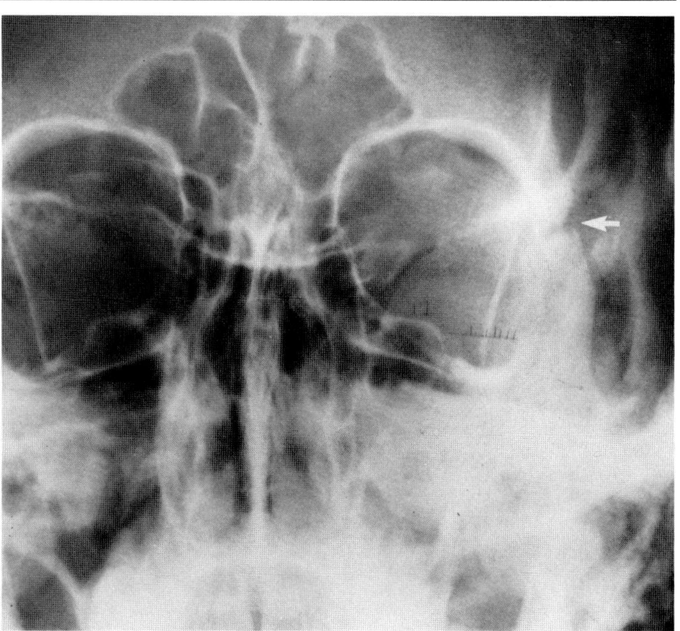

Figure 37B. The Caldwell view shows a zygomaticofrontal suture separation at arrow.

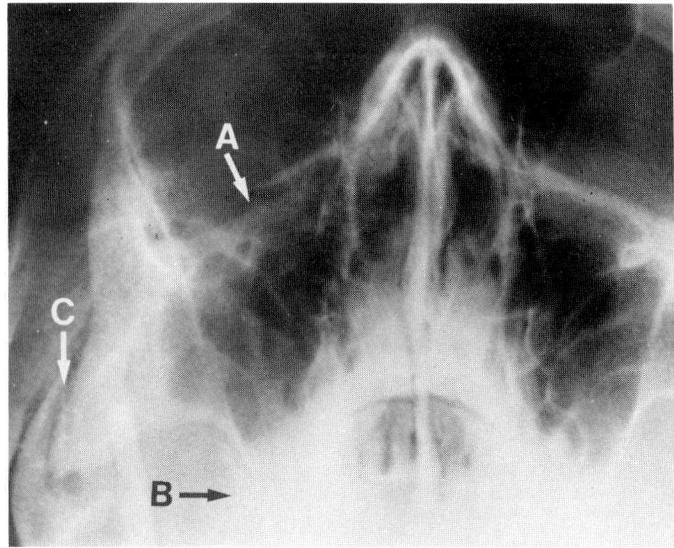

Figure 38A. Downward displacement of a right tripod fracture. Waters view showing low position of the outer rim fragment at A. Duplication of the lateral maxillary border at B. Downward zygoma fragment displacement at C.

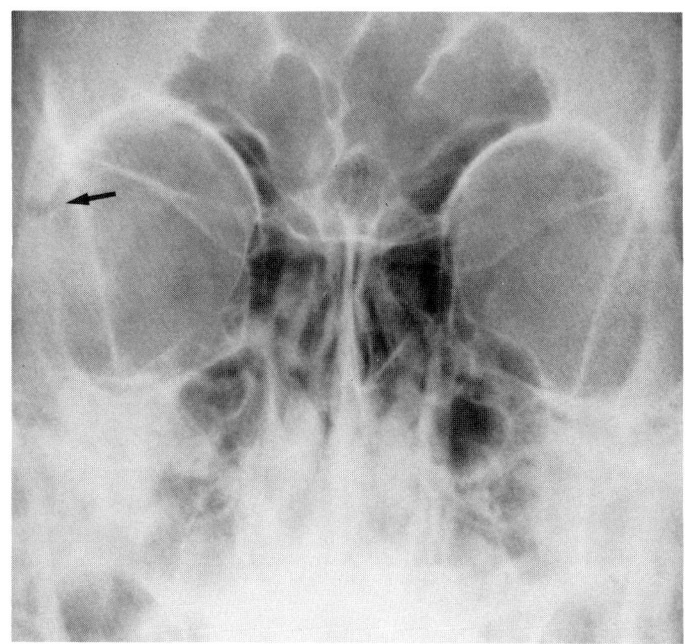

Figure 38B. Zygomaticofrontal suture separation at arrow.

Downward displacement of the movable anterior zygomatic arch fragment has also occurred.

Greater zygomaticofrontal suture separation is present on the Caldwell view in Figure 38B.

After reduction, the orbital rim and zygomaticofrontal fixation points produced by wire sutures are illustrated in Figures 38C and D. Improved zygomatic arch and lateral maxillary wall fragment position is also present in these views.

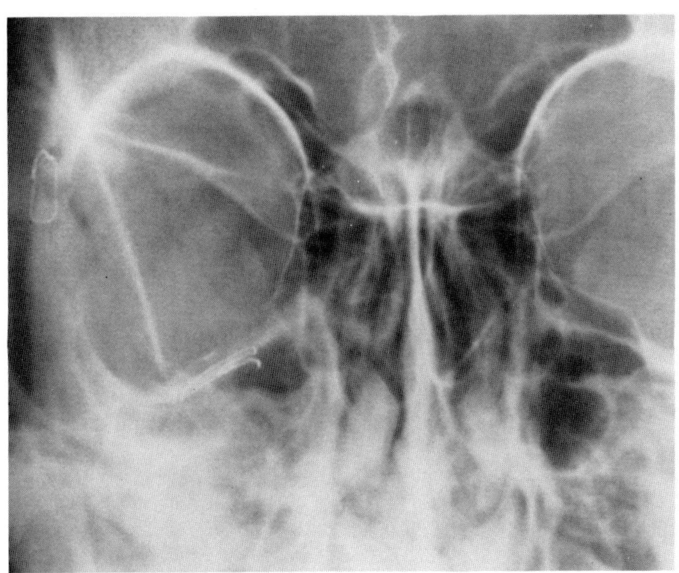

Figure 38C. Postreduction with orbital rim and zygomaticofrontal fixation wires on Waters view.

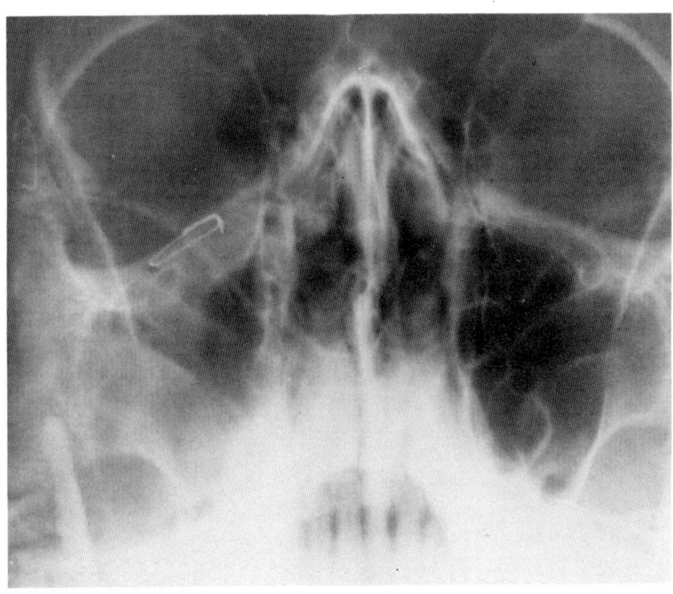

Figure 38D. Postreduction Caldwell view.

A. Supplementary Radiographic Views

We have seen how valuable the Waters and Caldwell views are in evaluating the tripod fracture.

The right tripod fracture illustrated by a Waters view in Figure 39A is barely visible due to minimal displacement.

A Towne projection of the same patient allows evaluation of the anterior, posterolateral, and medial maxillary sinus walls as seen in Figure 39B. On the patient's left, the sinus margins are intact. On the right, extensive comminution of the anterior and posterolateral maxillary surfaces as well as posterior displacement of the zygoma are present. The zygomatic arch is usually too overexposed to view on a Towne projection, but may be seen on an underexposed projection.

We prefer the underexposed basal view to evaluate the zygomatic arch position and expect to obtain information about the zygoma body position as well.

A left tripod fracture is evident on the Waters view in Figure 40A. In this, a zygomatic arch interruption might be suspected from the angulation of the arch, but separation is not seen. The underexposed basal view (Figures 40B and C) clearly shows outbending of the zygomatic arch and also demonstrates posterior displacement of the zygoma body. One can also see that the left maxillary lateral incisor tooth is also missing, presumably as a result of the same fist fight that produced the tripod fracture.

The anterior and posterior maxillary portions as well as the zygomatic arch part of a tripod fracture is demonstrated in Figure 40D. In this axial CT view of the midmaxilla, a subtle separation of the anterior maxillary wall is present. Some comminution of the posterior maxillary wall is seen. Separation

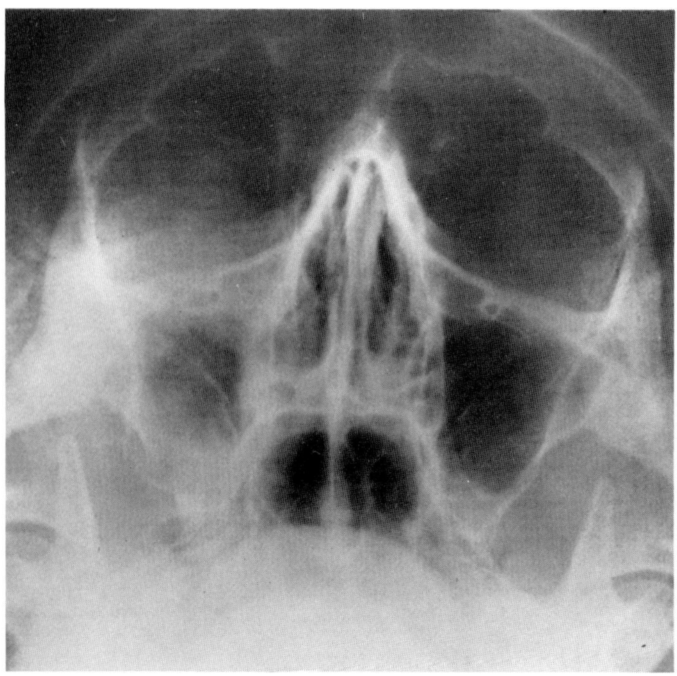

Figure 39A. The Towne projection in tripod fracture evaluation. Waters view with barely discernable right tripod fracture.

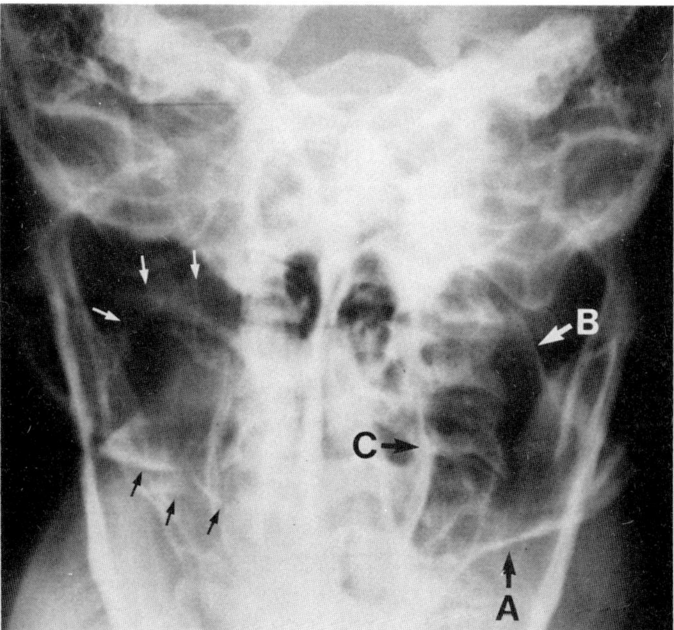

Figure 39B. Towne projection with intact anterior at A, posterolateral at B, and medial at C; maxillary margins on the left. Comminuted anterior and posterolateral margins on the right at arrows.

of the middle of the zygomatic arch is present. A small air-fluid level and a blood clot are evident in the maxillary sinus. Higher CT cuts (not illustrated) would be necessary to define the lateral orbital wall and zygomaticomaxillary suture interruption.

Polytomography and CT are reserved for evaluation of complications of the tripod fracture which are discussed in a subsequent section.

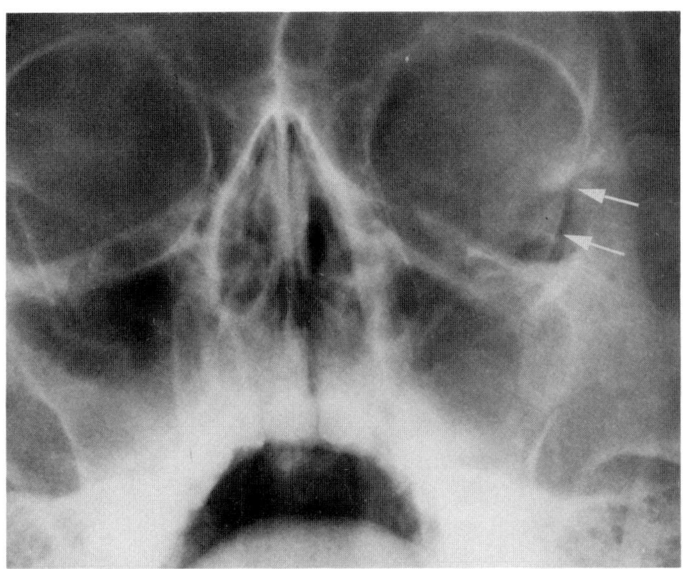

Figure 40A. Left tripod fracture. A Waters view clearly shows the fracture. A separation line parallels the left oblique orbital line.

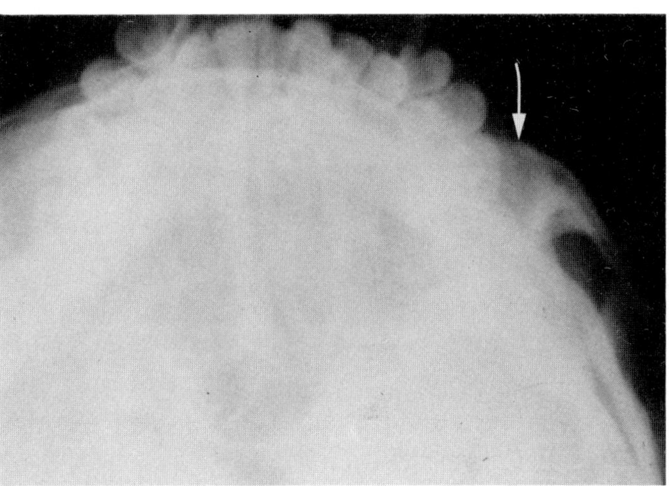

Figure 40B. An underexposed basal view.

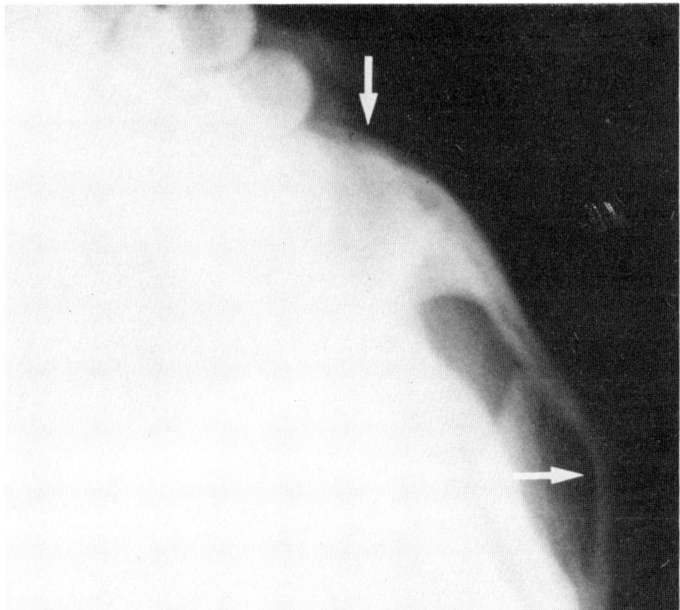

Figure 40C. Detail view of Figure 40B shows outbending of the zygomatic arch (horizontal arrow) and posterior displacement of the zygoma body (vertical arrow) when compared with the opposite side.

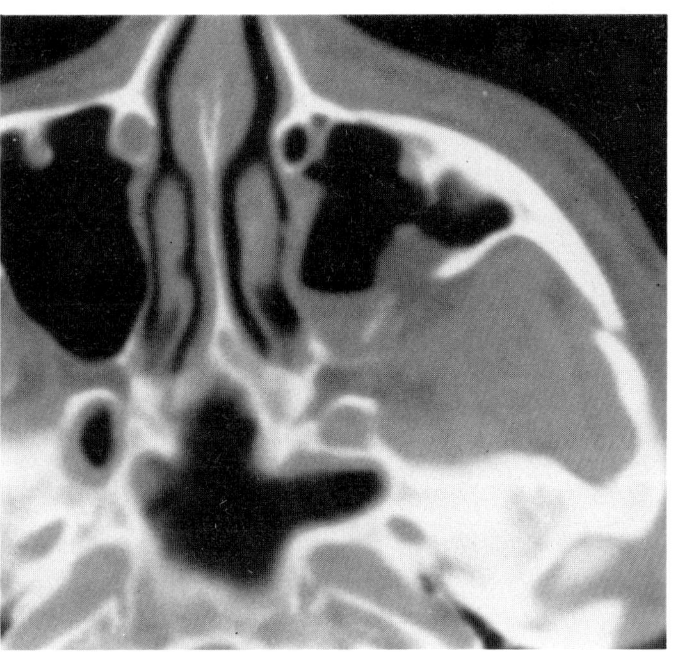

Figure 40D. A midmaxillary axial CT shows the anterior and posterior maxillary wall fractures and zygomatic arch interruption associated with a tripod fracture.

B. Mandibular Function

When the zygomatic arch portion of a tripod fracture extends into the glenoid fossa of the temporomandibular joint, mandible pain may restrict motion and simulate a mandibular condyle injury. The joint capsule may also be injured.

Occasionally, the tripod fragment may be so displaced that mandible motion is restricted. The zygoma fragment in Figure 41A is displaced downward to such an extent that it rests against the coronoid process of the mandible and prevents the patient from closing her mouth. The Caldwell view of this patient in Figure 41B best shows the amount of downward displacement of the tripod. This patient also has fractures of the nasal arch, frontal process of the maxilla, and the left maxillary alveolus. The alveolar injury produces the oblique position of the upper teeth seen in these views.

Inability to close the mouth implies injury while the mouth was open. Inability to open the mouth implies injury while the mouth is closed. This happened to the patient in Figure 42, where the zygoma was interposed against the coronoid process, and the patient could not open his mouth.

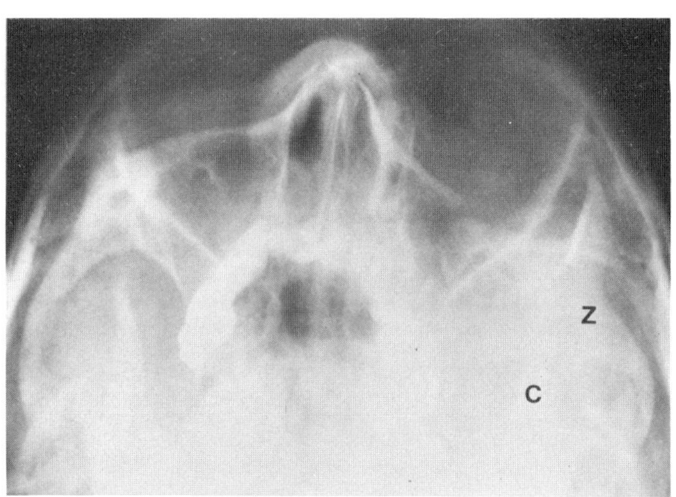

Figure 41A. Tripod injury and displacement preventing closure of mouth. Waters view with zygoma on coronoid process of mandible. Nasal arch and frontal process of maxilla are also fractured.

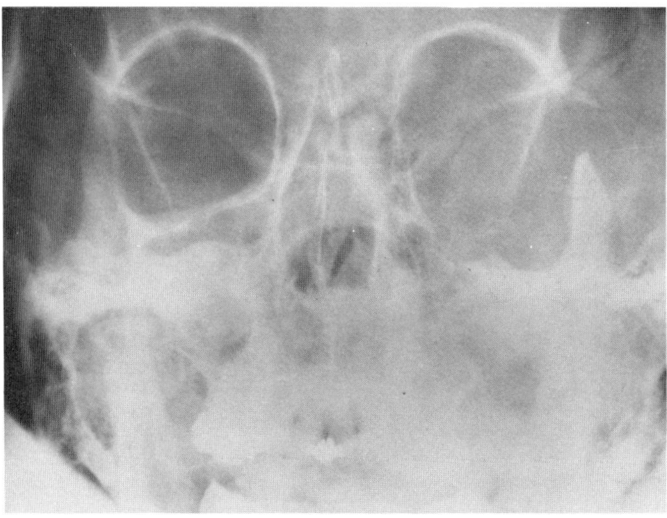

Figure 41B. Caldwell view with marked zygoma displacement.

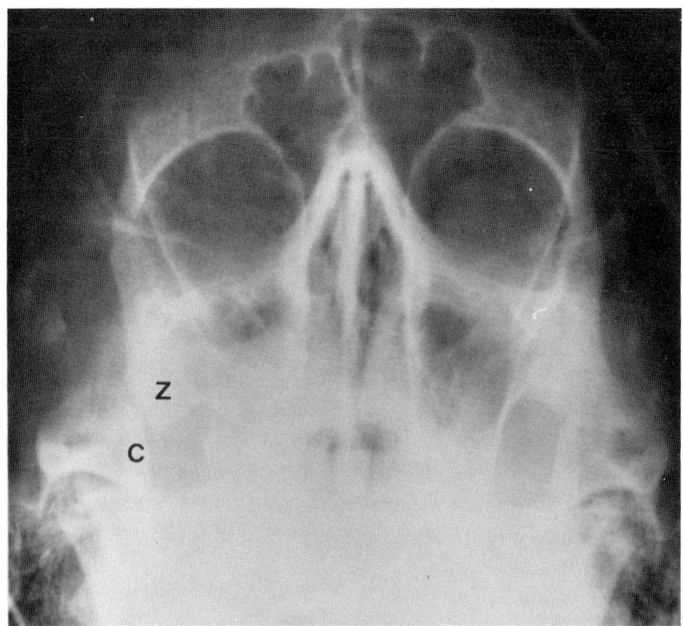

Figure 42. Zygoma displaced against the coronoid process preventing opening of mouth. Waters view.

C. Mandible Condyle Injury

The force that produces zygoma injury may also be applied to the mandible as might occur in the case of a fist-fight. Local mandibular fractures may be produced at the contact point of such a blow. Similarly, the mandibular force may be transmitted to the homolateral or contralateral mandibular neck or condyle. The condyle may be displaced into the tympanic bone, which forms the posterior wall of the glenoid fossa. The result may be a mandible neck fracture, a mandible condyle fracture, a tympanic bone fracture, or some combination injury of these parts.

The temporal bone examination in Figure 43 ("B") shows the combination of a mandible condyle and tympanic bone fracture. This axial CT is an oblique axial view through the external auditory canal and glenoid fossa. The condyle was displaced posteriorly against the tympanic bone, was sheared off of the

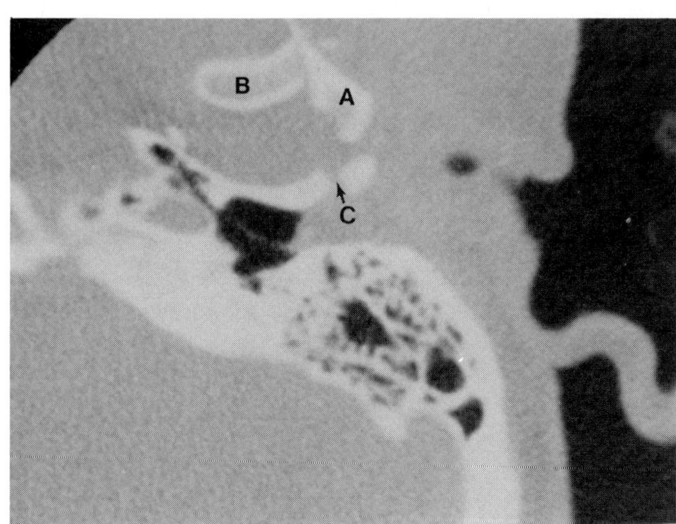

Figure 43. Axial CT of the left temporal bone. (Anterior direction is upward.) A. Mandible neck. B. Mandible condyle fragment from the medial part of A. C. Tympanic bone fracture.

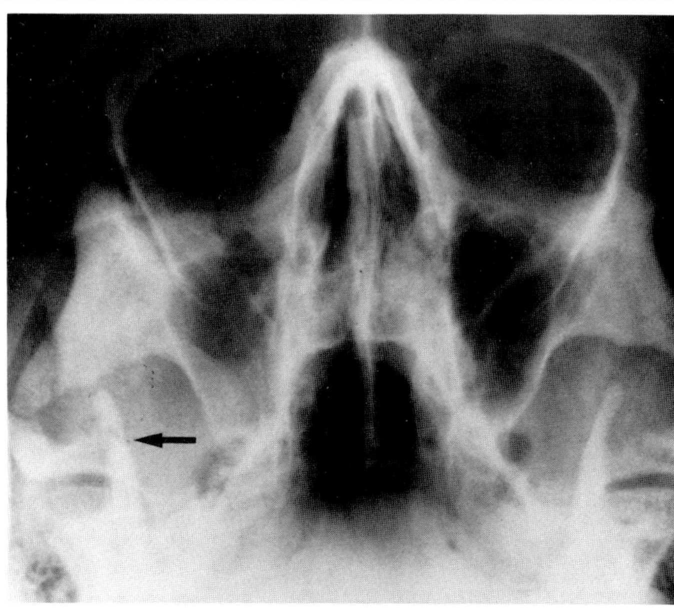

Figure 44. Right tripod and fracture of coronoid tip (arrow).

mandible neck, and was displaced out of the glenoid fossa indicating injury to the mandibular capsule. The posterior displacement of the mandible neck sheared off the most peripheral portion of the tympanic bone. A hematoma accompanying the tympanic fracture fills the external auditory canal. Absence of blood in the middle ear space and mastoid indicates that there is no involvement of the temporal bones. The patient did have conductive hearing loss due to the external auditory canal hematoma.

The patient illustrated in Figure 44 had a shearing fracture of the coronoid process tip secondary to the displacement of a tripod fracture.

A mandible ramus fracture may also be produced during the same altercation that results in a tripod fracture. Such an injury is demonstrated in Figure 45 in which a left tripod fracture is present in the Waters view (Figure 45A). A posteroanterior view, Figure 45B, shows the accompanying intercondylar mandible fracture.

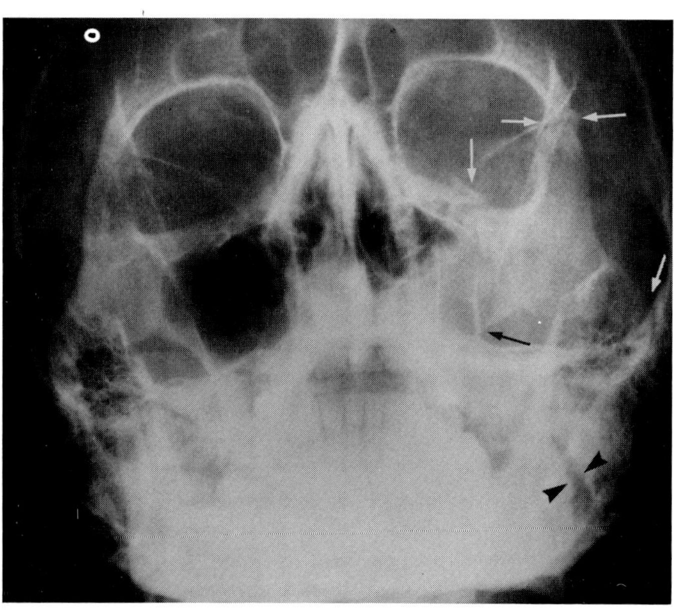

Figure 45A. Left zygoma and mandible fractures. Waters view of the left tripod fracture. Mandible fracture at arrowhead.

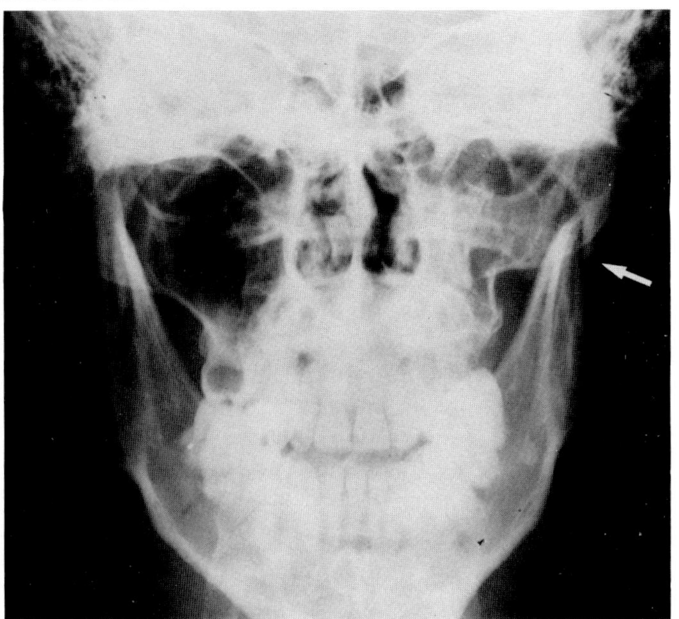

Figure 45B. Posteroanterior view with intercondylar fracture at arrow.

D. Variations in Lateral Orbital Involvement

While the majority of tripod fractures involve the zygomaticofrontal suture, variations in fracture position occur and require adjustments in the surgical repair.

The orbital process of the zygoma is interrupted in Figure 46A. The zygomaticofrontal suture is intact. Orbital process fixation was produced with a suture spanning the fracture as seen in Figure 46B.

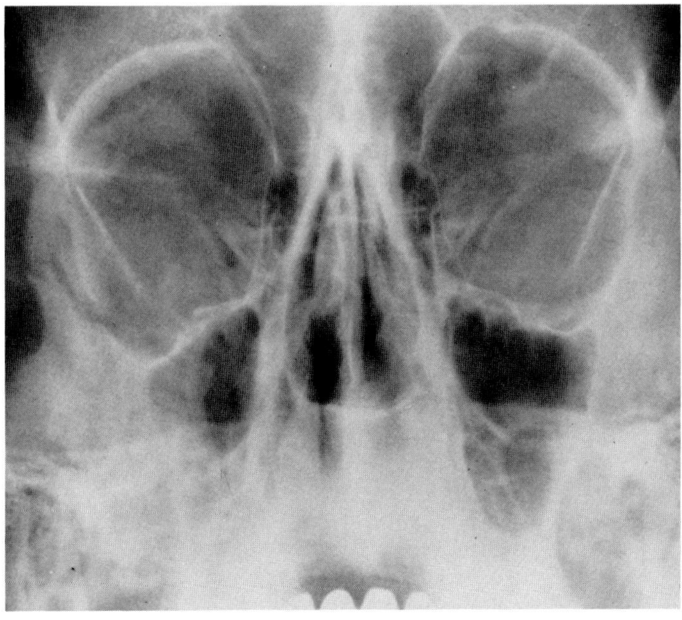

Figure 46A. Low-lying orbital process fracture. Preoperative view.

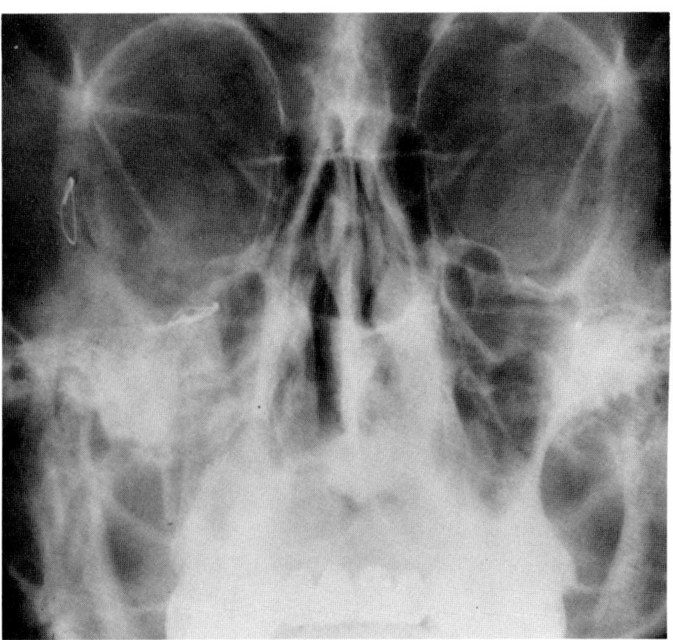

Figure 46B. Postoperative view.

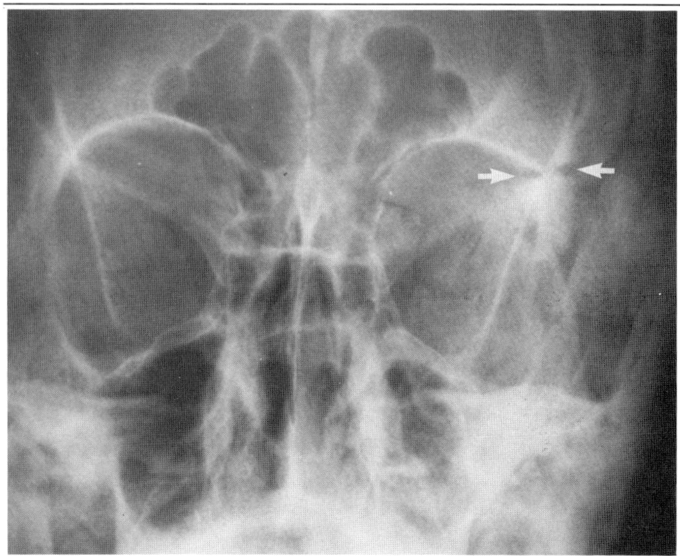

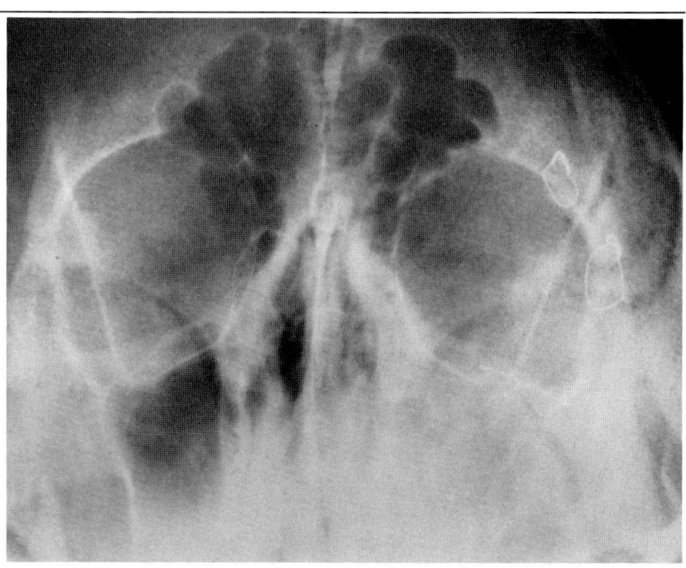

Figure 47A. High orbital process fracture. Preoperative view with fracture through the base of the orbital process of the frontal bone.

Figure 47B. Postoperative view.

The orbital process of the frontal bone may be sheared off in association with a tripod fracture. When this occurs, there is usually accompanying separation of the zygomaticofrontal suture as well. This is seen in Figure 47A where medial displacement of both the zygomatic and frontal contributions to the lateral orbital wall are present. The surgeon, again, must adjust the suture fixation points to produce stability as evident in Figure 47B.

Medial displacement of the orbital process is usually accompanied by extensive orbital floor injury as seen in Figure 48A. The transverse orbital dimension is markedly narrowed by the displaced orbital process of the

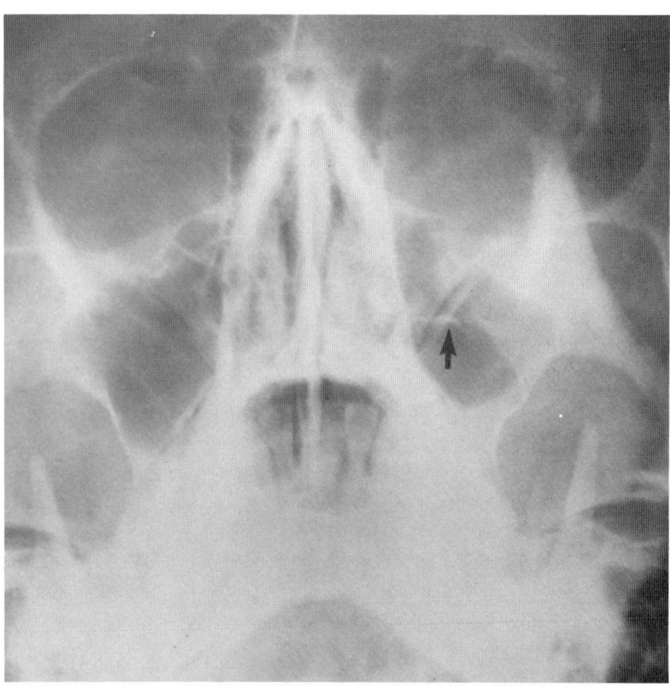

Figure 48A. Medial displacement of the lateral orbital border with orbital floor interruption. Waters view. Displaced orbital floor at arrow.

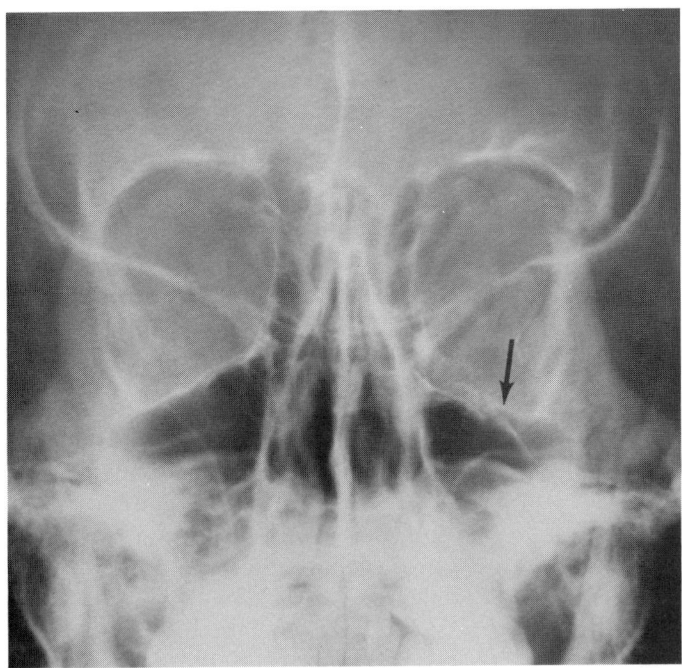

Figure 48B. Caldwell view with comminuted orbital floor at arrow.

zygoma. The comminuted orbital floor is displaced into the maxillary sinus in Figure 48B. Clinically, no ocular muscle entrapment was present, but lateral gaze was restricted.

If the greater wing portion of the lateral orbital border is injured, the oblique orbital line will be interrupted, and an overlap sign will appear where fragments are superimposed as in Figure 49A. The fragment superimposition is best defined on axial CT examination as illustrated in Figure 49B.

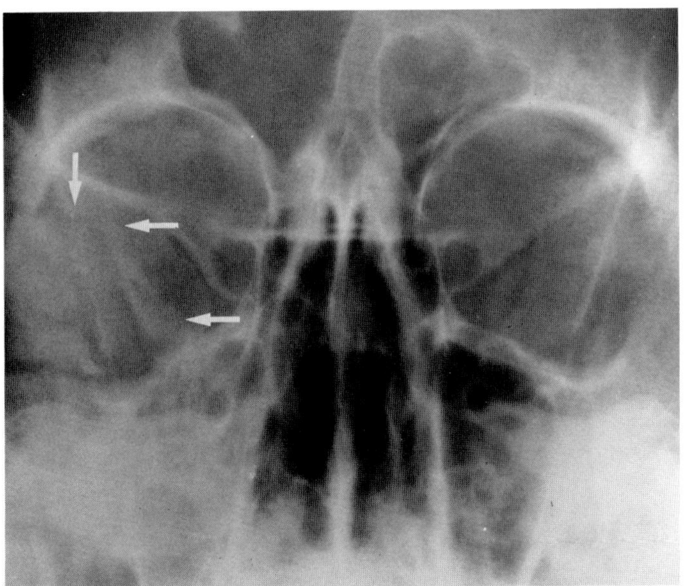

Figure 49A. Right tripod fracture with injury of orbital process of greater wing. Caldwell view with OOL interruption at vertical arrow and overlap sign,at horizontal arrows.

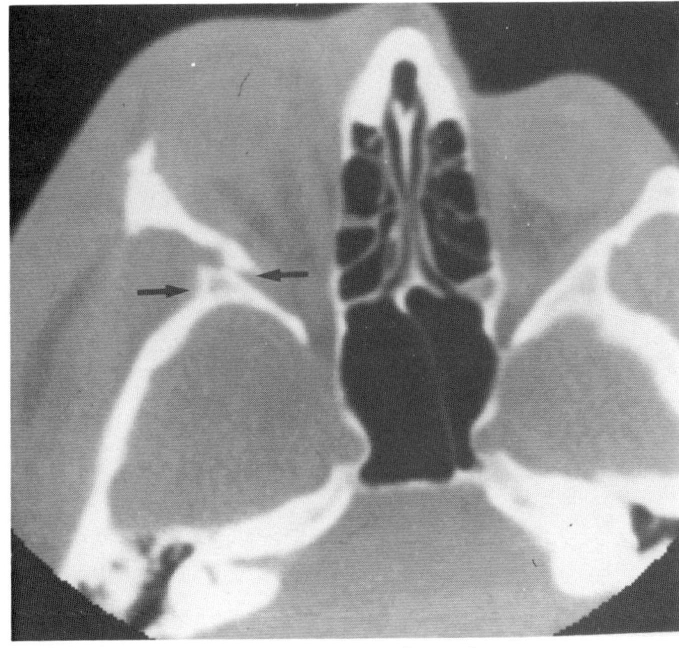

Figure 49B. Axial transorbital CT with overlap at arrows.

E. Orbital Apex and Optic Canal Injury Complicating the Tripod Fracture

If the force producing a tripod fracture is directed along the long axis of the lateral orbital wall, injury to the orbit apex and surrounding structures may occur. We use tomography and CT to demonstrate suspected orbital apex injury.

The patient illustrated by Figure 50 had a right tripod fracture accompanied by diminished vision in the right eye. Careful evaluation of the Caldwell view revealed an abnormal linear density along the lateral border of the superior orbital fissure (Figure 50A). A view from the coronal tomographic study confirmed the greater wing fracture and demonstrated a lesser sphenoidal wing fracture with clockwise rotatory displacement (Figure 50B). Ethmoidal sinus opacity is also present on the right.

In Figure 51, another patient with a right tripod fracture and orbital apex injury is shown. Figure 51A is a coronal polytomogram illustrating a lesser wing fracture with clockwise rotation similar to that in Figure 50B. The lateral tomograms, in Figures 51B and 51C, show how the lesser wing and anterior clinoid process have been separated from the planum sphenoidale and tuberculum sellae.

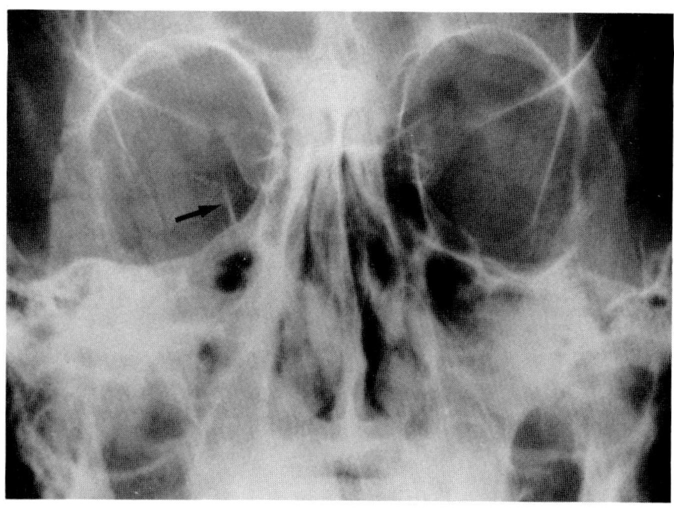

Figure 50A. Right tripod fracture with orbital apex injury. Caldwell view with abnormal linear density at arrow.

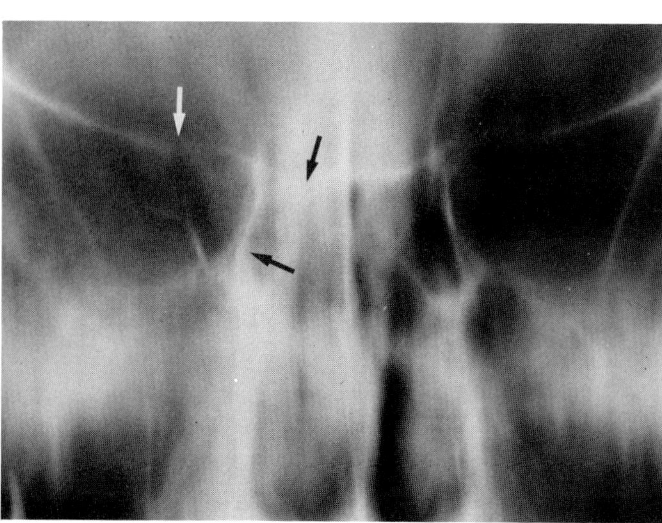

Figure 50B. Coronal tomograph of superior fissure area. Clockwise rotation of lesser sphenoidal wing with fractures at arrows.

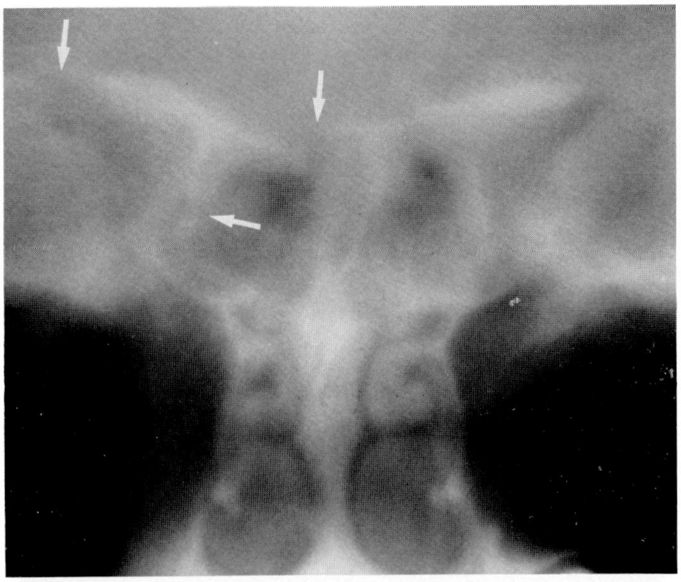

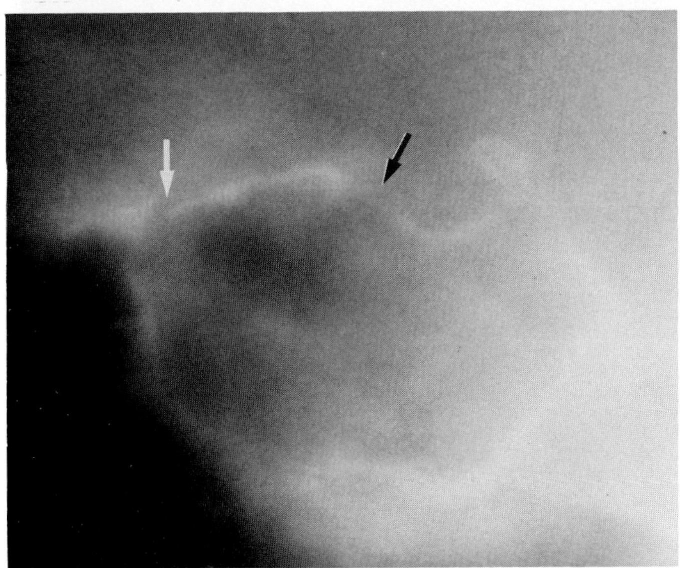

Figure 51A. Right tripod fracture with orbital apex injury. Rotated lesser wing with fractures at arrows on coronal polytomogram.

Figure 51B. Lateral sella polytomogram with lesser wing separation at arrows.

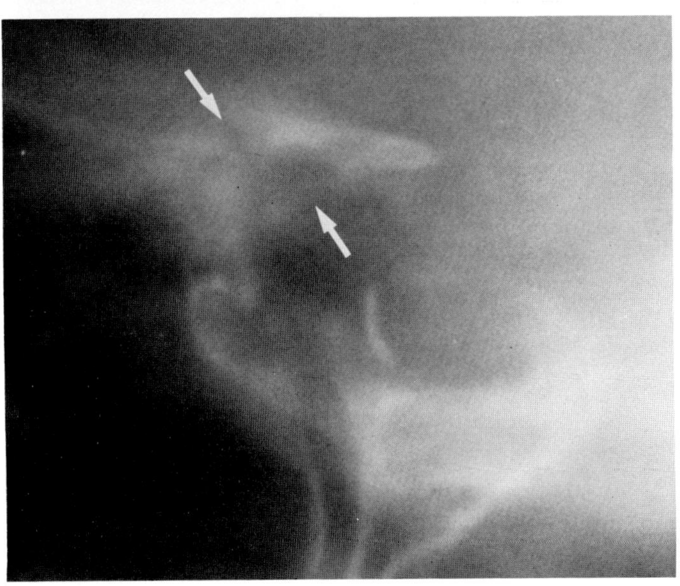

Figure 51C. Lateral parasellar polytomogram with lesser wing and anterior clinoid separation at arrows.

A CT study of a similar injury is demonstrated by Figure 52. Figure 52A is a transmaxillary axial view showing interruption of the left anterior and posterolateral maxillary borders. In Figure 52B, the plane is through the midorbit. Angulated fragments of the orbital process of the greater sphenoidal wing have been displaced into the orbital apex. Ethmoidal and sphenoidal sinus opacity imply medial orbital wall injury. A coronal CT reconstruction shows how the greater wing border of the superior fissure has been displaced upward above the lesser wing (Figure 52C). This markedly narrows the superior orbital fissure.

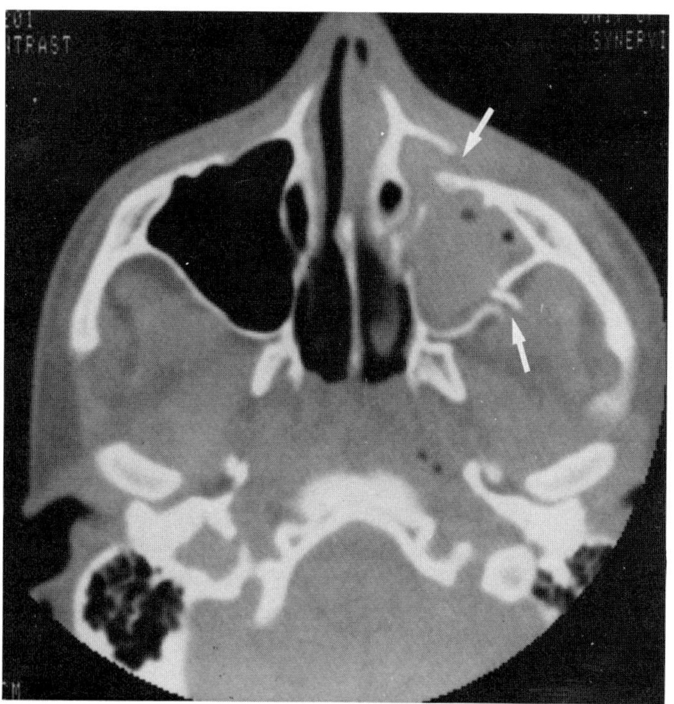

Figure 52A. Left tripod fracture with orbital apex injury. Transmaxillary CT with anterior and posterolateral maxillary fractures at arrows.

Figure 52B. Transorbital CT with displaced fragments of the orbital process of greater wing. The fragment at A would produce an abnormal linear density area on plain films.

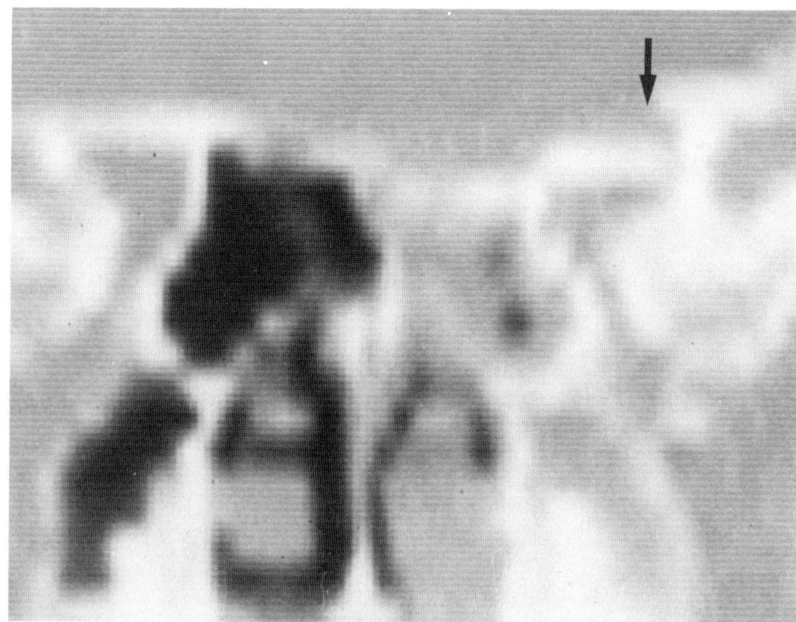

Figure 52C. Elevated greater wing at arrow on coronal CT reconstruction.

This case demonstrates combined tripod and orbital apex injury resulting from a force directed through the tripod, the lateral orbit wall, and into the orbit apex. The orbital apex injury may also result from a force directed from the lateral toward the medial portion of the orbit.

Lateral compression producing a right maxillary wall interruption is evident in the axial CT of Figure 53A. These fractures are typical of those found in a tripod fracture. A lateral blow is indicated by the medial displacement of

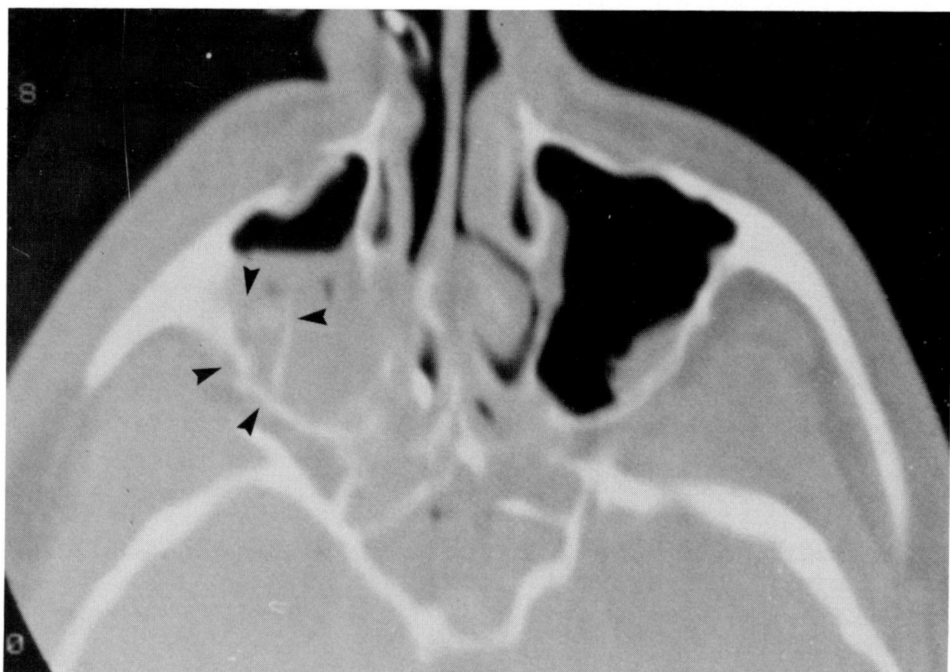

Figure 53A. Lateral compressive force producing a tripod fracture and orbital apex fractures. An axial midmaxillary CT shows maxillary wall fractures typical of a tripod injury (arrowheads). Medial displacement of the right zygoma is present, and similar compression of the right sphenoidal surface of the middle temporal fossa is present.

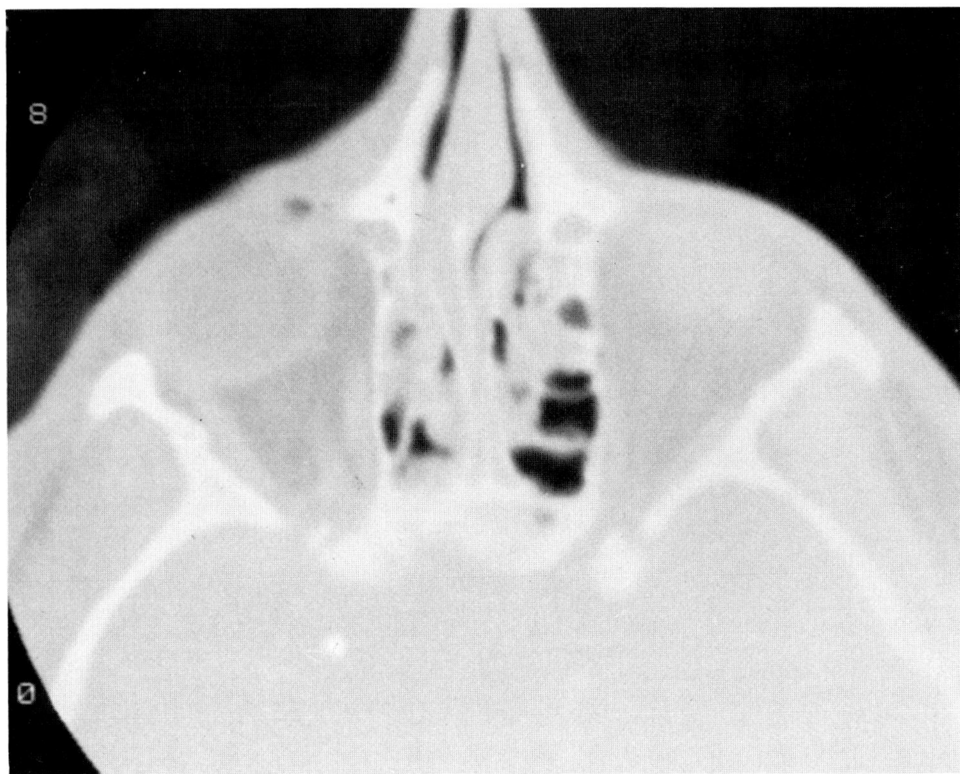

Figure 53B. A higher midorbit CT reveals a right lateral orbit wall fracture, lamina papyracea compressive flattening, and comminution of the anterior clinoid and adjacent sphenoidal surface of the right optic canal.

the zygoma body into the maxillary sinus. Compressive change from the right lateral direction has also displaced the bony border of the right temporal fossa so that this side is smaller in size than the left temporal fossa.

A higher axial midorbit cut is shown in Figure 53B. In this illustration, a fracture of the lateral orbital wall through the base of the sphenoid orbital process is present and the lateral orbital wall is displaced medially. Lamina papyracea flattening is present and resulted from compression of the orbital soft tissue content against the ethmoid surface. This view also reveals comminution of the right anterior clinoid process and the sphenoidal margin of the optic canal, which also resulted from lateral compressive force.

Sometimes the tripod fracture is only an incidental shearing component of a more significant injury along the upper orbit and frontal sinus as seen in Figure 54.

A Waters view of this injury, Figure 54A, shows primarily a left tripod fracture with slight caudal displacement of the fragment. The Caldwell view, Figure 54B, reveals a comminuted fracture involving the left orbit upper rim and roof, the frontal sinus walls, glabella, and left lamina papyracea. The right side is intact. This injury pattern indicates that the left frontal and orbital region was the contact area, while the left tripod complex was merely sheared and shifted by the force application.

CT examination of the upper orbital rim and frontal sinus revealed details of the injury in this area. Figure 54C illustrates the depression of a large anterior frontal fragment into the frontal sinus and upper orbit. A higher axial CT, Figure 54D, demonstrates comminution in the area of the lateral orbital roof. Extensive damage of the frontal sinus and orbit roof in an injury such

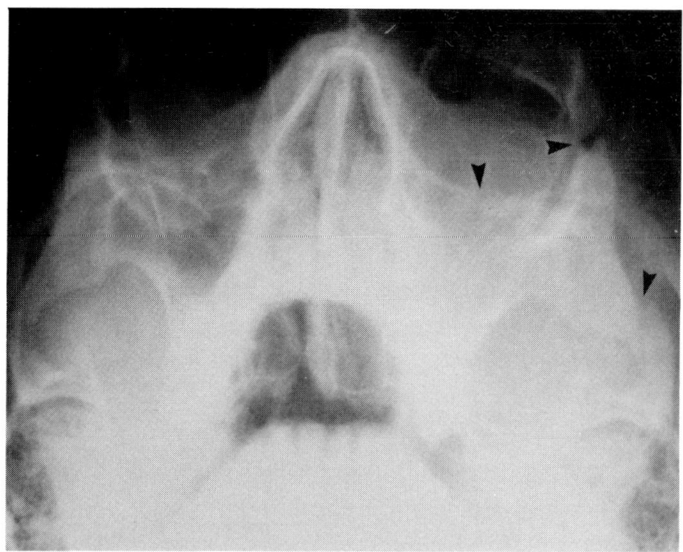

Figure 54A. Primary upper orbit rim and frontal sinus injury with incidental tripod fracture. Waters view with left tripod fracture (arrowheads).

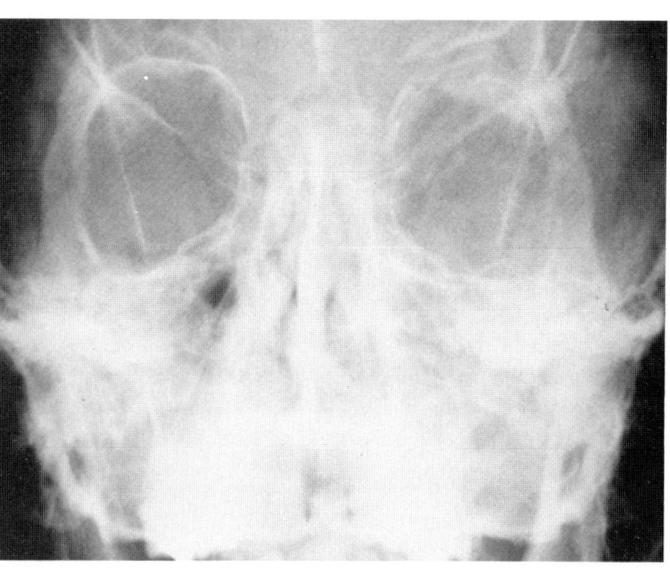

Figure 54B. Caldwell view revealing extensive left upper orbit rim and roof fracture and involvement of the frontal sinus walls, glabella, and lamina papyracea fractures.

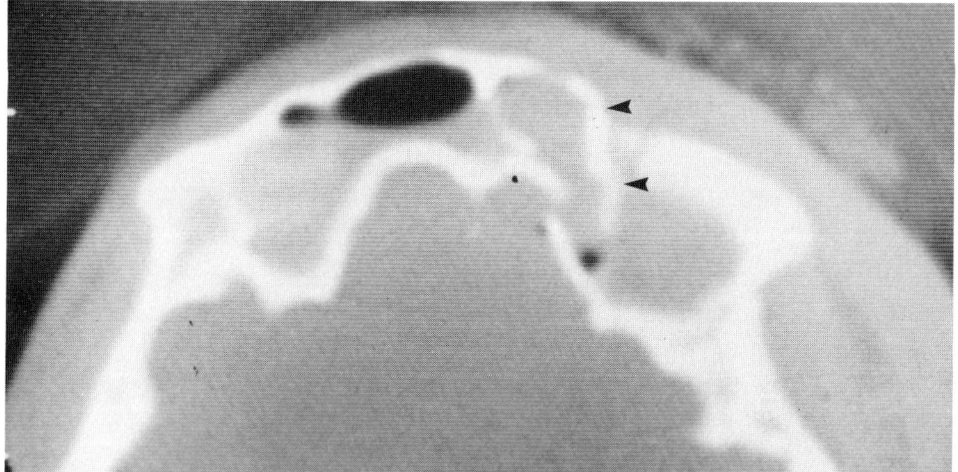

Figure 54C. Axial CT of upper orbit and frontal sinus. Large depressed left frontal sinus anterior wall fracture depressed into the sinus and upper orbit (arrowheads).

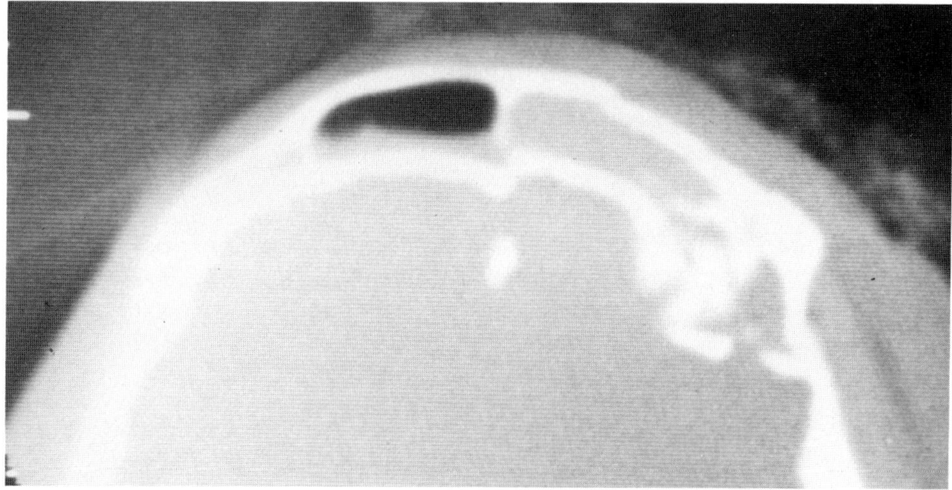

Figure 54D. Higher axial CT to show the comminuted lateral orbital roof.

as this would specifically indicate the presence of underlying anterior fossa meningeal and brain injury.

Thus, the tripod fracture can vary from a relatively minor, isolated fracture producing flattening of the malar eminence to an incidental finding in association with other injury that can imperil vision or be associated with significant meningeal or brain injury. One should not stop evaluation with discovery of a tripod fracture, but should be very careful to evaluate surrounding structures that may also be involved in a given injury.

F. Bilateral Tripod Fracture

On occasion, a patient may have a tripod fracture on both sides as seen in Figure 55A. The examiner must make sure that the central nasal-frontal axis is not injured in order to differentiate the bilateral tripod injury from the more extensive LeFort II injury form.

The Caldwell view, Figure 55B, shows zygomaticofrontal suture separation on the left, while the right orbital process has a transverse fracture below the suture.

Fixation sutures following fracture reduction are shown in Figure 55C.

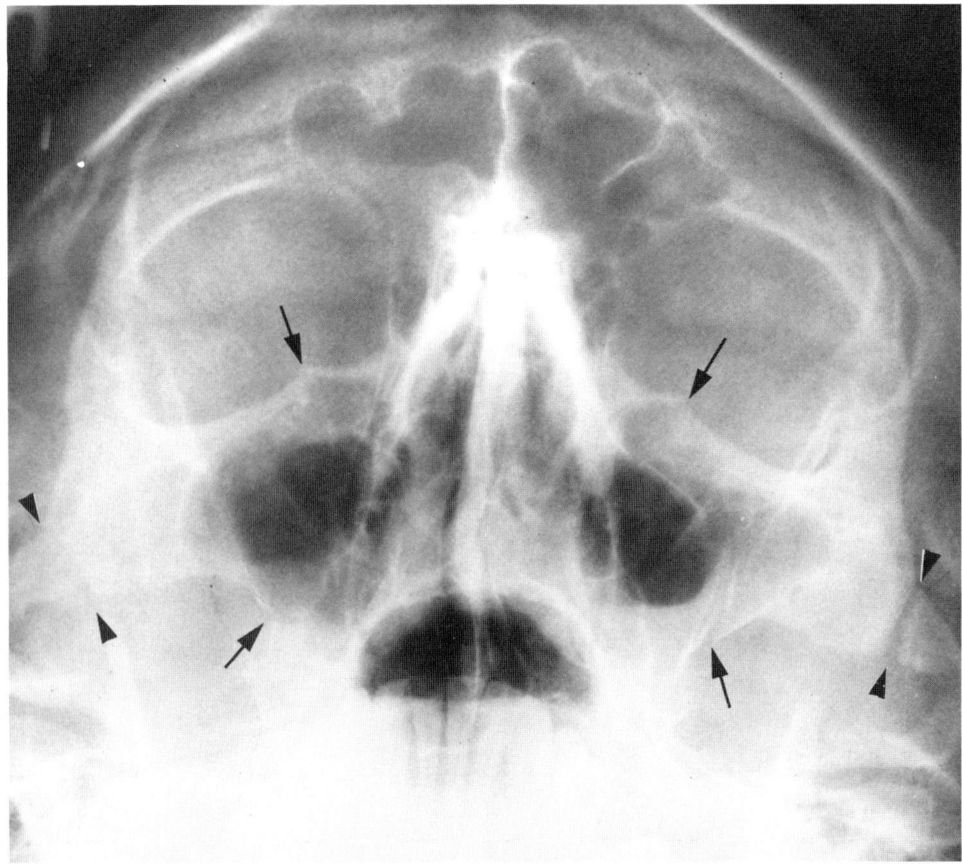

Figure 55A. Bilateral tripod fractures. Waters view shows the transmaxillary and arch fractures.

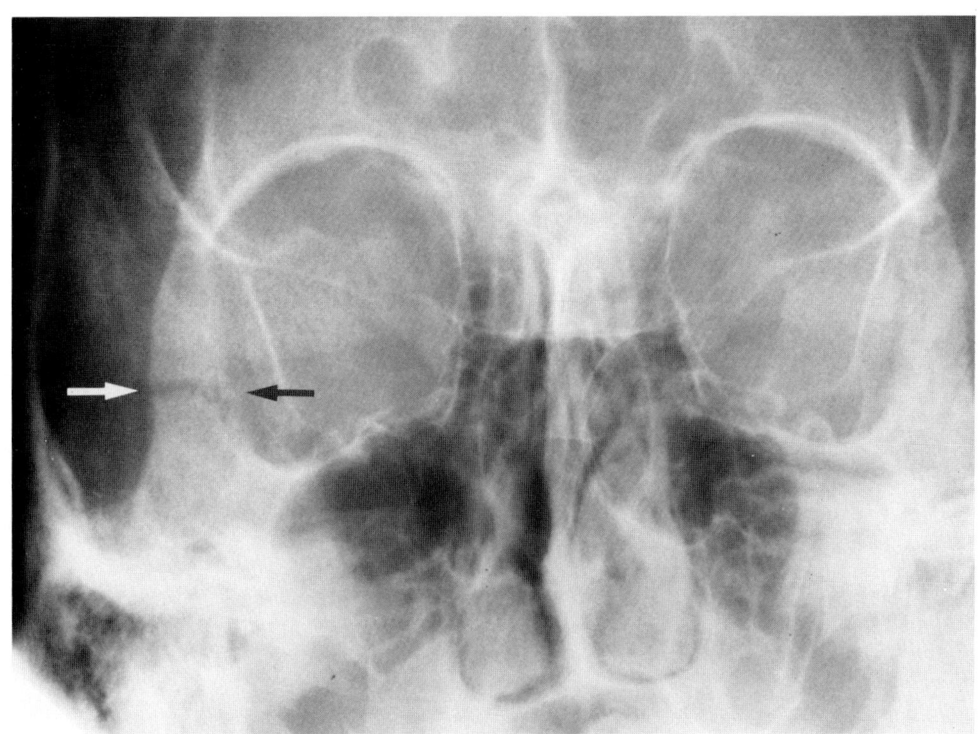

Figure 55B. The zygomaticofrontal suture is separated on the left, while a transverse orbital process fracture (arrows) is present on the right in the Caldwell view.

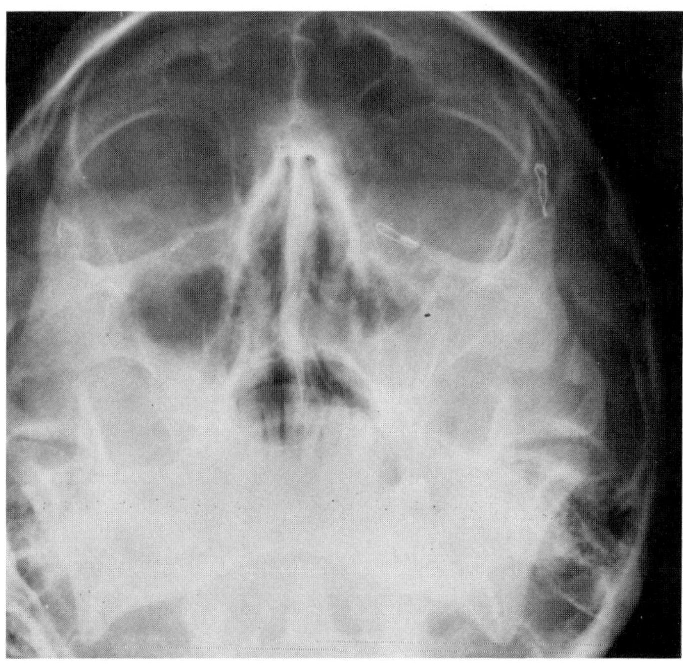

Figure 55C. Post reduction and fixation Waters projection.

2. FRONTAL PROCESS OF MAXILLA INJURIES

As seen in the Waters view in Figures 3A and 3B, the frontal process of the maxilla is a structure that when paired with the opposite side forms the lateral bone boundaries of the nasal pyramidal below the nasal bones. The Caldwell view in Figures 2A and 2B demonstrate how the frontal process extends upward just posterolateral to the nasal bones. This portion behind the nasal bones joins the frontal bone just below the glabella.

Along the medial wall of the orbit, the frontal process of the maxilla lies posterior to the nasal bones and immediately anterior to the lacrimal fossa. The posterior frontal process edge forms the anterior margin of the lacrimal fossa, while the lacrimal bone forms the floor of the lacrimal fossa proper.

A fracture separating the frontal process of the maxilla from the surrounding attachments may occur in association with severe nasal bone injury as described previously. This process may also be fractured along with the tripod by a frontal blow.

The patient whose examination is illustrated in Figure 56 was injured in an car accident. The frontal process is fractured along with the nasal arch on both sides, and a left tripod fracture is also present.

The transmaxillary axial CT section in Figure 56A demonstrates a left tripod fracture with posterior and lateral displacement of this fragment. The left frontal process and subadjacent lacrimal bone canal have been separated from their maxillary attachments and displaced posteriorly when compared with the right side, which is normal in position. Fractures of the frontal process lamella lying alongside of the nasal fossa, as well as the perpendicular ethmoid plate, are present and slightly displaced. Subcutaneous air and soft tissue swelling are present anterior to the left maxillary sinus surface. The left maxillary sinus and nasal fossa are opaque due to a blood accumulation.

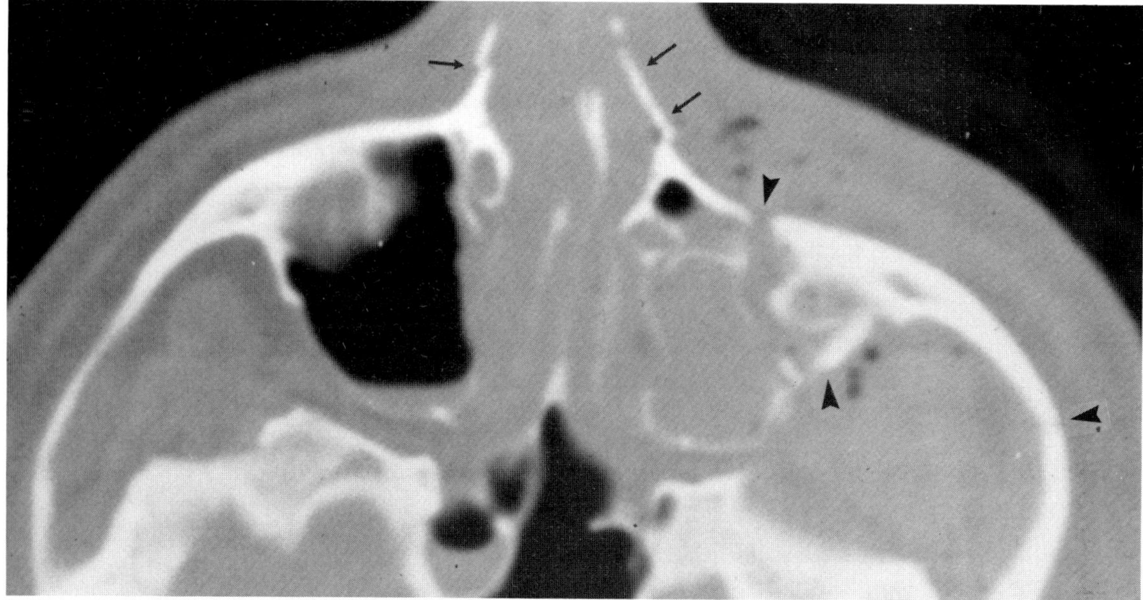

Figure 56A. Axial CT examination of a left tripod fracture associated with frontal process of maxilla and nasal arch fractures. Midmaxillary plane showing maxillary and zygomatic components of a tripod fracture (arrowheads). The left frontal process is depressed, and the lamella of both frontal processes is fractured (arrows).

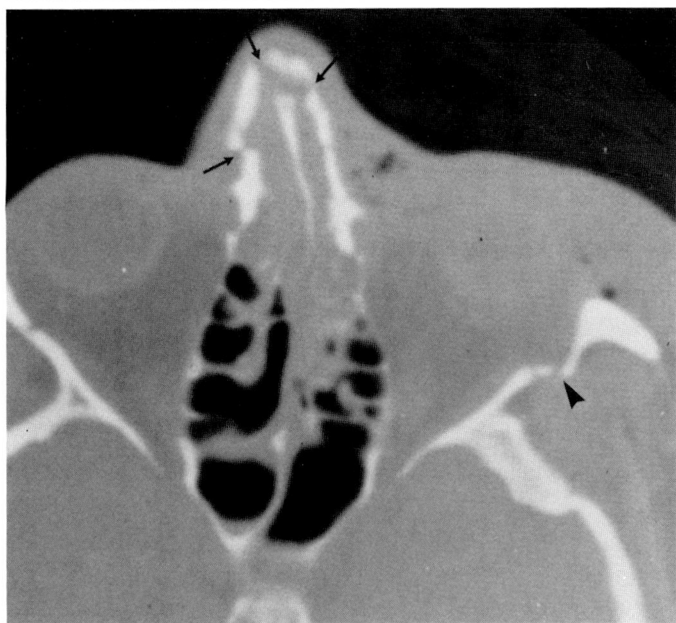

Figure 56B. A midorbit section shows a fracture through the zygomatic process of the lateral orbit (arrowhead). Nasal arch and frontal process comminution is present centrally (arrows). The left lacrimal fossa is displaced posteriorly into the ethmoid sinus.

A nasal arch comminuted fracture highlights the midorbit axial CT in Figure 56B. Separation of the lacrimal fossa edges from surrounding structures is also present. The left lacrimal bone margins have been displaced posteriorly into the anterior ethmoid sinus cells producing opacity, while several posterior ethmoid sinus cells are clear as is the sphenoidal sinus. A fracture of the zygomatic orbital process with lateral displacement is also present and completes the tripod portion of this fracture. Prominent periorbital and malar soft tissue swelling is present.

An axial CT view in the plane of the upper orbit and the glabella is demonstrated by Figure 56C. In this section, the highest level of the frontal

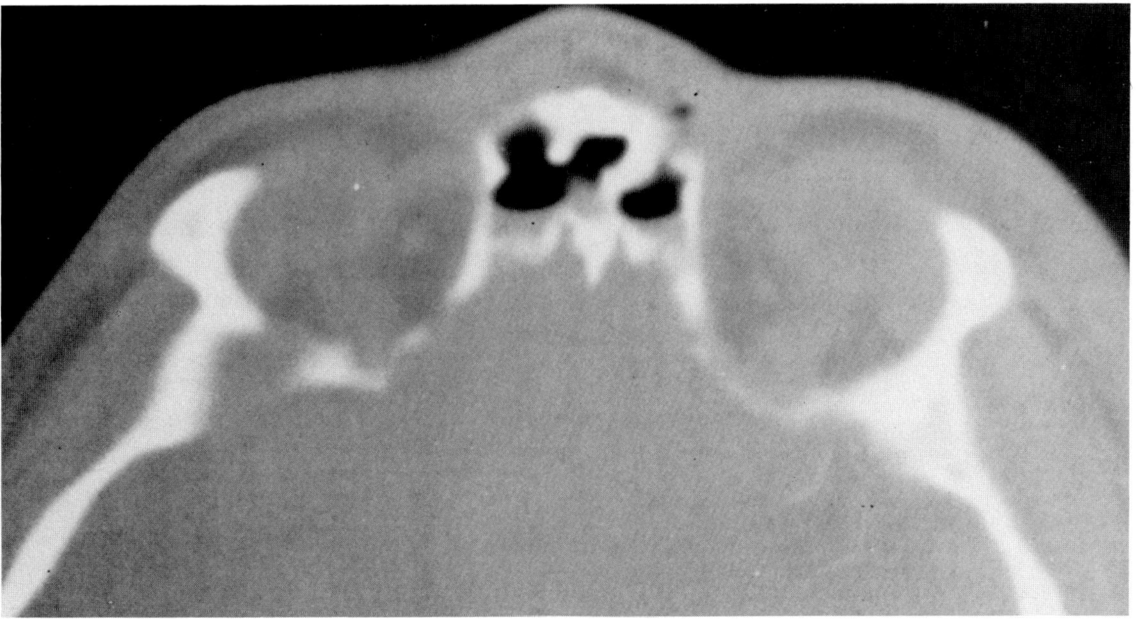

Figure 56C. A high orbit view showing the top of the left frontal process (arrow) next to the intact glabella. The lateral orbital wall is intact.

process fracture on the left is shown. The glabella is intact, and the lateral orbital process of the frontal bone is also intact. This case illustrates the close relationship between the frontal process of the maxilla and the lacrimal fossa and bony canal.

Serious injury to the lacrimal sac, contained in the fossa, or to the lacrimal duct within the bone canal, can be associated with injury of the frontal process. Such an injury can cause epiphora, which may also be produced by simple periorbital soft tissue swelling. The epiphora produced by soft tissue swelling usually decreases and disappears as the swelling decreases. Dacrocystography by contrast or isotope examination may be needed to show the location of a block in persistant epiphora.

Bilateral frontal process comminution, severe nasal arch fractures and lacrimal canal fractures are illustrated in Figure 57. This injury also resulted from a car accident.

The Waters plain film in Figure 57A shows bilateral maxillary air-fluid levels. The medial inferior orbit borders are fractured and displaced downward on both sides, while the lateral inferior orbit border, zygoma, and zygomatic arches are intact. The nasal arch and both maxillary frontal processes are interrupted. The orbit floor has also been displaced downward on both sides and lies just above the air-fluid level.

CT examination confirmed the plain film findings and demonstrated further details of the lacrimal bone canal details. Figure 57B, an upper maxilla section, shows the anterior maxillary wall fractures on both sides. A fracture of the medial attachment of the frontal process through the lacrimal canal is also present bilaterally. The canal fragments on the left side have also been compressed to produce narrowing that distorts the canal shape.

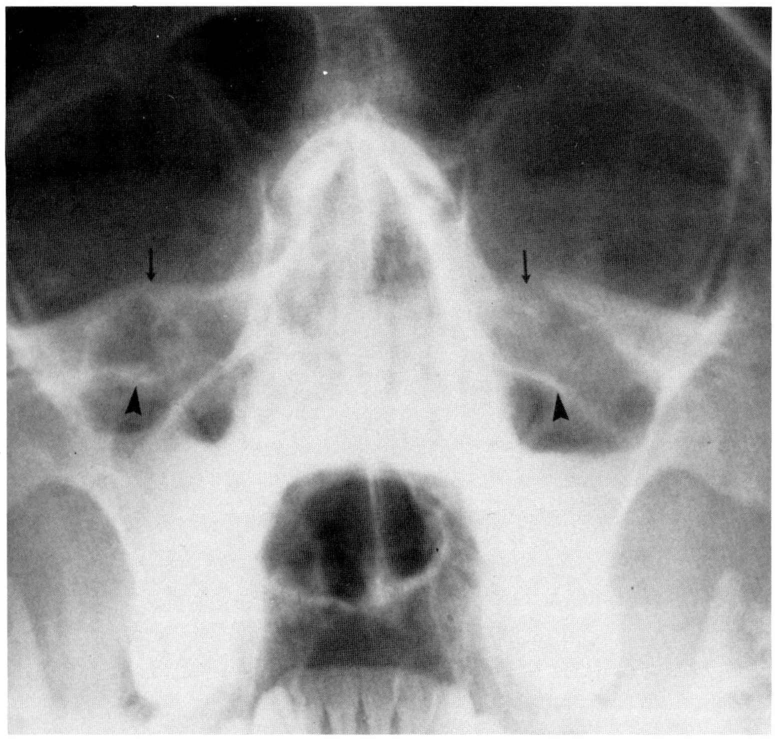

Figure 57A. Examination of an injury producing bilateral frontal process, nasal arch, and marked lacrimal fossa and canal fractures. A Waters view with bilateral air-fluid levels. Fractures interrupt the medial lower orbit rims, the frontal processes, and the nasal arch (arrows). Downward displacement of both orbit floors is present (arrowheads).

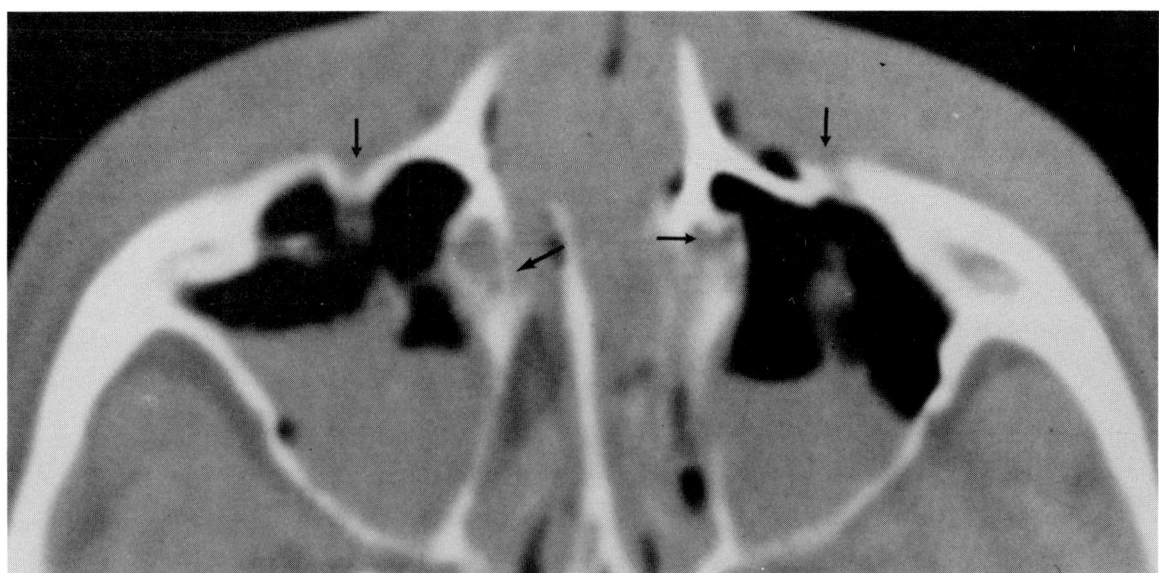

Figure 57B. Midmaxillary axial CT with anterior maxillary wall fractures and medial wall fractures through the lacrimal bone canals (arrows). The zygomatic arches are intact.

A view made 6 mm higher through the lower orbit, Figure 57C, shows compressive change of both frontal processes, which have been driven posteriorly into the lacrimal fossa and ethmoid sinuses. The lamellae of both frontal processes are fractured, and extensive periocular air surrounds the globe on both sides.

An upper orbital section in Figure 57D shows the nasal arch comminuted fracture accompanied by interorbital soft tissue swelling. Higher cuts showed no evidence of glabella or frontal sinus fracture (not illustrated).

This case demonstrates maximal central injury that may be associated with a frontal process of maxilla fracture. As shown, the tripod fracture is not necessarily present with a frontal process injury. Usually, the presence of a tripod fracture implies that the force producing the frontal process injury

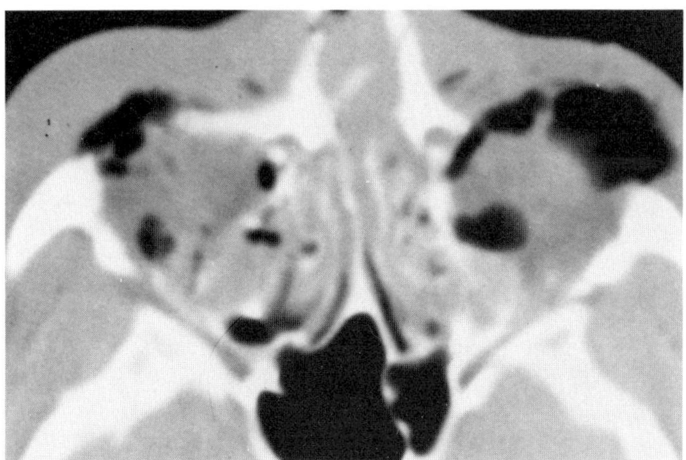

Figure 57C. Lower orbit axial CT with frontal process depression that distorts the lacrimal bone fossae. Extensive periocular air is present.

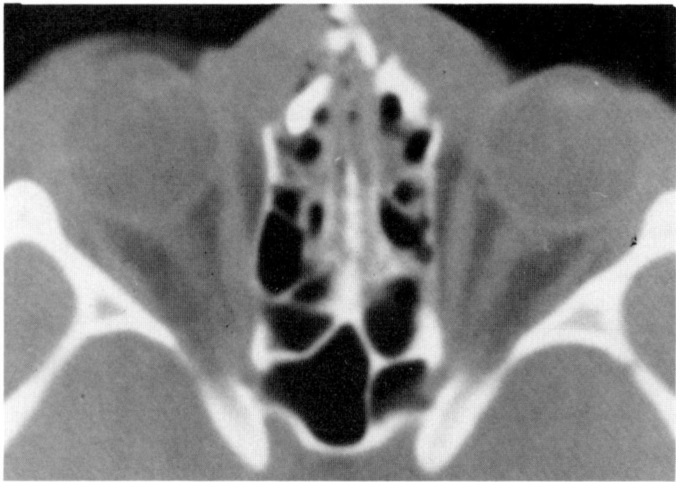

Figure 57D. A higher axial transorbit view shows nasal arch comminution.

was slightly off center or that the object striking the face was broad enough to shear off the tripod, as well as to produce the frontal process fracture.

Thus far, the fracture patterns we have presented affect only a local portion of the facial skeleton. Perpendicular or horizontal buttresses may be interrupted on one side, but the facial skeleton fragment is comparatively small.

Usually, the force producing local fractures is relatively small so that the collective facial bones are not affected. A few cases such as that illustrated by Figure 56 show two distinct areas of injury, the central nasal skeleton and the peripheral tripod fragment. However, in this injury the opposite side was not seriously injured.

Greater forces produce local comminuted fractures at the point of contact with the facial skeleton and have sufficient shearing force on the facial skeleton so that the perpendicular or horizontal buttresses on both sides are also fractured resulting in large facial fracture fragment. The large fragment may be divided into one or more component fragments. The resulting injury form can best be described as a "complex fracture."

5
Complex Injuries

Complex facial injuries are either bilateral or imply severe comminution of several parts of the facial bone complex. We divide this category of injury into the LeFort and "smash" types of fracture.

1. LeFORT INJURIES

René LeFort was a French surgeon who extensively studied severe facial injury and who produced essentially three facial injury forms in the laboratory. His articles have been translated by Tilson, McFee, and Soudah (see suggestions for further reading).

From his experimental work, LeFort described three planes of injury that represent lines of "weakness" of the facial bones and result in separation of a large fragment after injury. This separation results in instability and altered position of the fragment. Treatment is aimed at restoring stability and functional position of the upper jaw.

LeFort's planes of weakness are outlined in Figure 58. Figure 58A is a depiction of LeFort lines in the Caldwell position; Figure 58B is a lateral view of the lines. In the lateral view, the LeFort III fracture crosses the lateral orbital wall and zygomatic arch. LeFort originally described the craniofacial separation as the first plane of weakness and the transmaxillary plane as last. For some reason, unknown to us, customary contemporary usage describes the transmaxillary fracture as the LeFort I and the craniofacial separation as the LeFort III fracture. To avoid confusion, we are using the contemporary designation.

A. LeFort I Fracture

The LeFort I plane of weakness traverses both medial and lateral walls of the maxillary sinuses. Posteriorly, the pterygoid processes of the sphenoid are interrupted. This results in a "floating palate" fragment. Often the maxillary

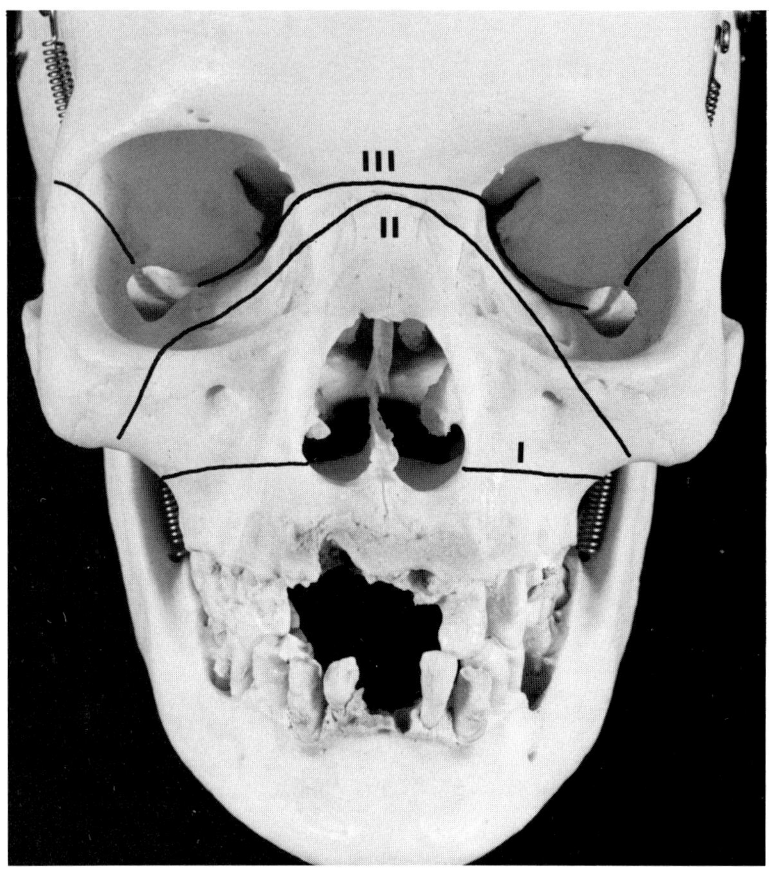

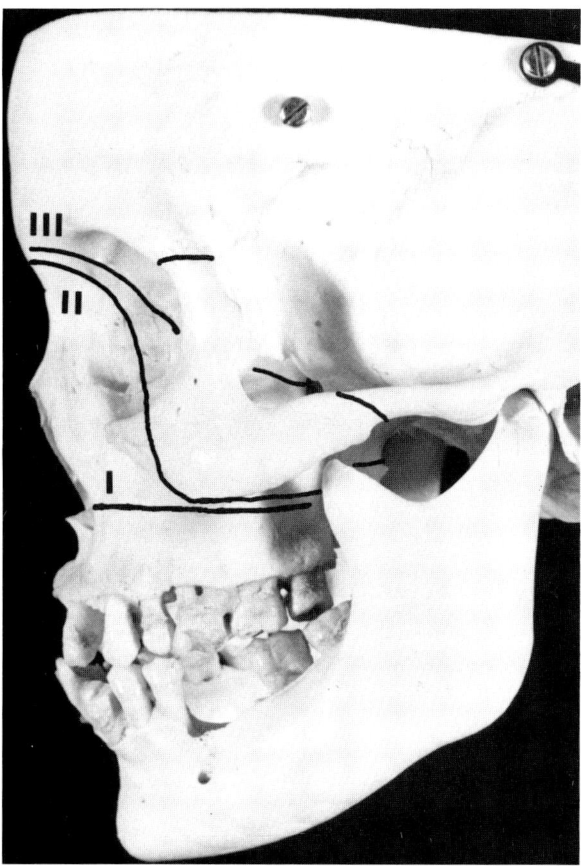

Figure 58A. The LeFort planes of weakness. Anteroposterior view.   **Figure 58B.** Lateral view.

dental arch will be in the "anterior open bite" position, in which the maxillary molars are approximated to the mandibular molar teeth while the incisors of both jaws are separated.

We begin evaluation of a LeFort injury with inspection of the lateral view, which allows evaluation of the pterygoid processes and posterior maxillary walls. In Figure 59A, the pterygoid processes are interrupted. Similarly, the walls of one zygomatic recess have been fractured. An anterior maxillary fracture separation is also present, as is a slight anterior open bite.

The transmaxillary fracture is best seen in the Waters view, Figure 59B. This also shows the anterior open bite and extension of the fracture through the inferior portion of the left zygomatic recess.

Restoration of dental structure position was accomplished with interdental wires. Further stabilization was produced by suspension wires placed through drill holes in the zygoma body as seen in Figure 59C. The suspension wires were attached to the interdental wires below. This brings the movable maxillary fragment into optimal position in respect to the stable portion of the maxilla as shown in Figure 59C.

Computerized tomography axial sections are helpful in evaluating the palatal injury resulting from a LeFort I injury. Not only is the palate separated from the vertical maxillary buttresses and pterygoid plates, but the palate may also be divided by the injuring force.

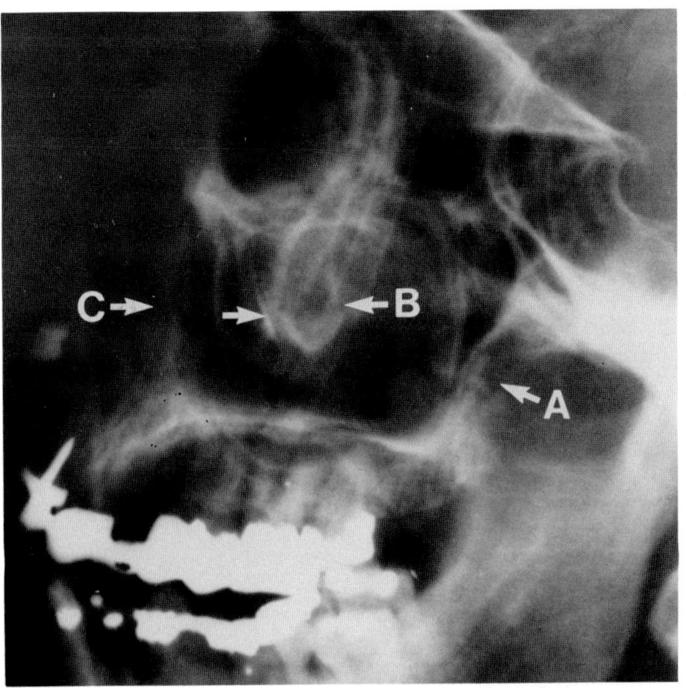

Figure 59A. LeFort I fracture. Lateral view with pterygoid process fractures at A, zygomatic recess fractures at B, and anterior maxillary surface fracture at C.

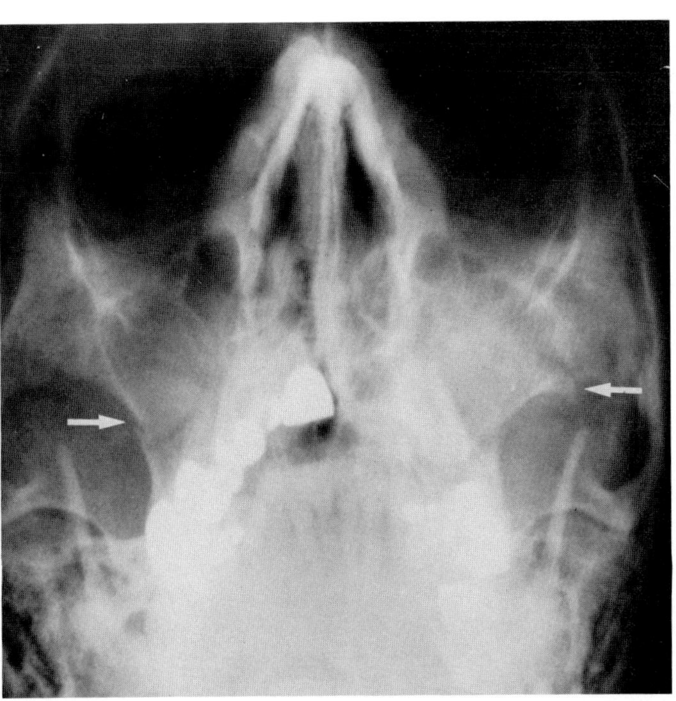

Figure 59B. Waters view showing transmaxillary fractures at arrows.

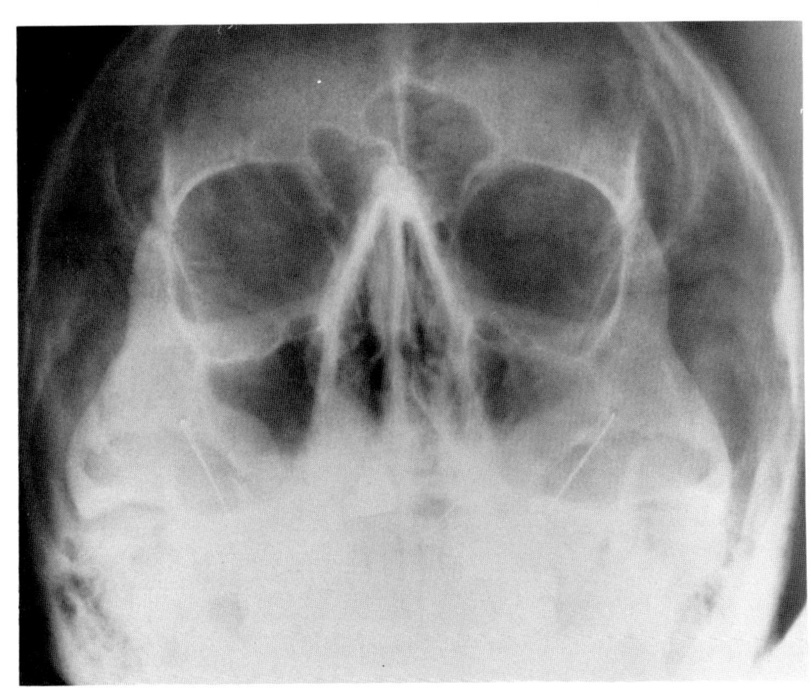

Figure 59C. Postreduction and suspension view.

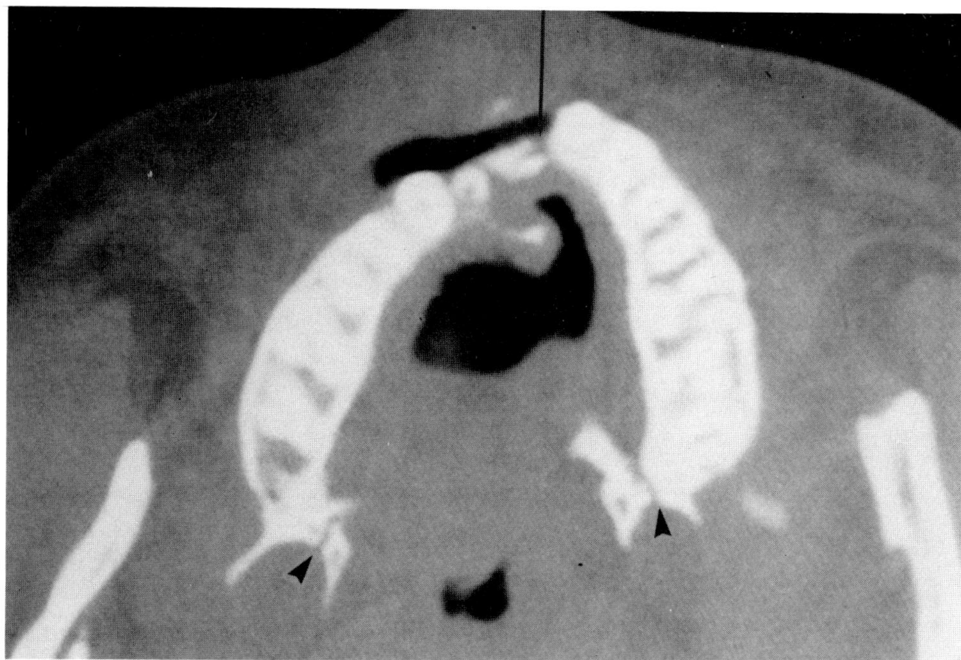

Figure 60A. LeFort I fracture on CT. Axial CT through the maxillary alveolus in a LeFort I injury. Alveolar separation present anteriorly (arrow). Pterygoid process fractures posteriorly (arrowheads).

Figure 60A is an axial CT section through the alveolar arch of a patient with a LeFort I fracture. Wide separation of the alveolar arch is present anteriorly where the fracturing force contacted this part. Posterior shearing force has driven the arch against the caudal pterygoid plates and interrupted them. The alveolar arch has been divided into two parts.

A slightly higher palatal alveolar section, Figure 60B, further illustrates the two alveolar arch fragments and their separation from the horizontal body

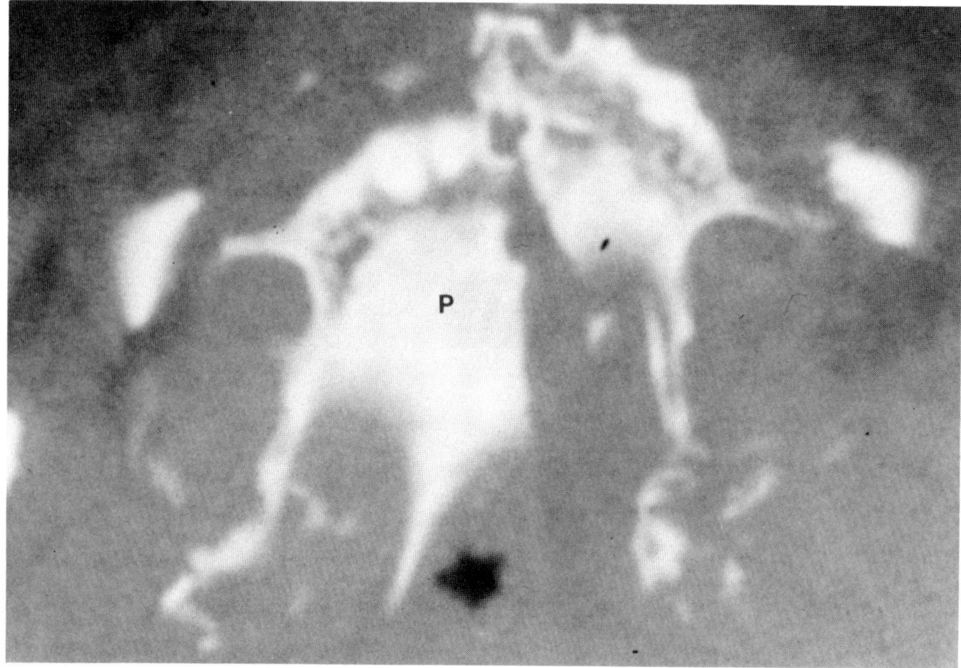

Figure 60B. Axial CT through the hard palate (P) in a LeFort I injury.

of the palate so that three fragments, the right maxillary alveolus, the left maxillary alveolus, and the hard palate, are separated from one another. Pterygoid plate fractures are again evident.

B. LeFort II Fracture

The LeFort II fracture illustrated by Figure 61A has interrupted the pterygomaxillary cortices. A slight posterior position of the palatal fragment is present. The margins of both zygomatic recesses of the maxillary sinus have been interrupted, and nasal-ethmoidal area comminution is present. A slight anterior open-bite position of dental structures is evident.

Downward displacement of the "pyramidal" fragment is illustrated by the Waters view in Figure 61B. The nasal arch and underlying glabella are fractured. Both inferior orbital borders are interrupted. A step-off is present on the right, while less displacement is present on the left. Both lateral maxillary walls are fractured at the inferior zygomatic margin and at the junction between the lateral maxillary wall and the dental alveolus.

Both lateral orbital walls and zygomatic arches are intact. The right frontal process of the maxilla is comminuted and rotated off axis so that it is not seen in this view (disappearing fragment sign). The left frontal process is in good position, but is separated from the medial maxillary wall. The left

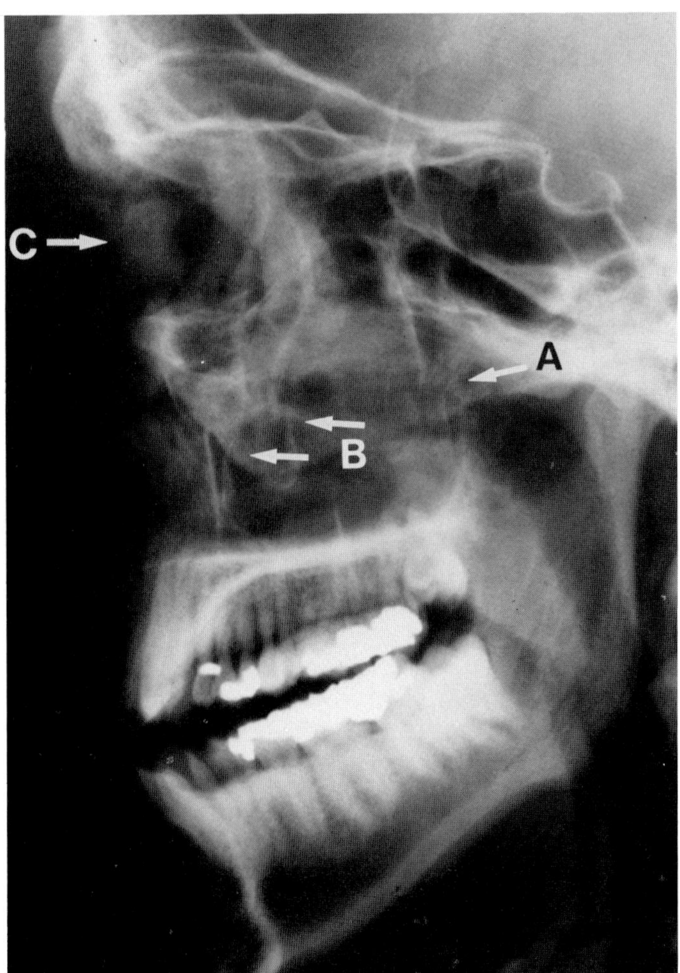

Figure 61A. LeFort II fracture. Lateral view with pterygoid process fractures at A, zygomatic recess fractures at B, and nasal-ethmoidal fracture at C. Note the posterior position of the hard palate and slight anterior open bite.

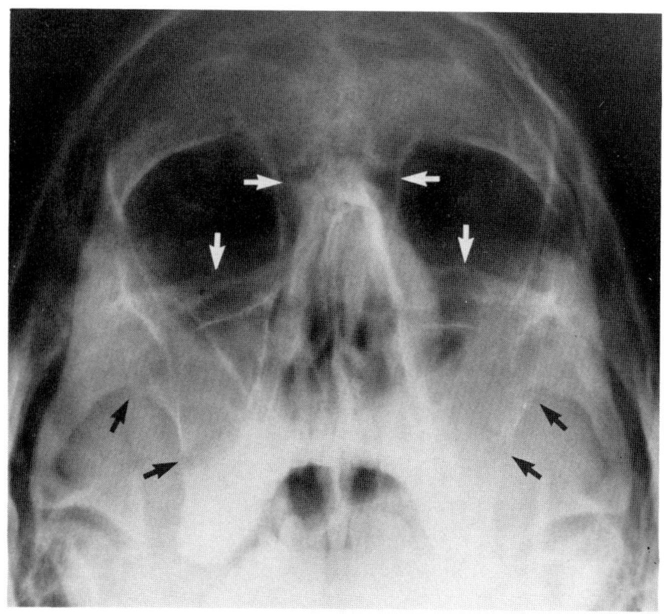

Figure 61B. Waters view showing pyramidal fragment produced by fractures at arrows.

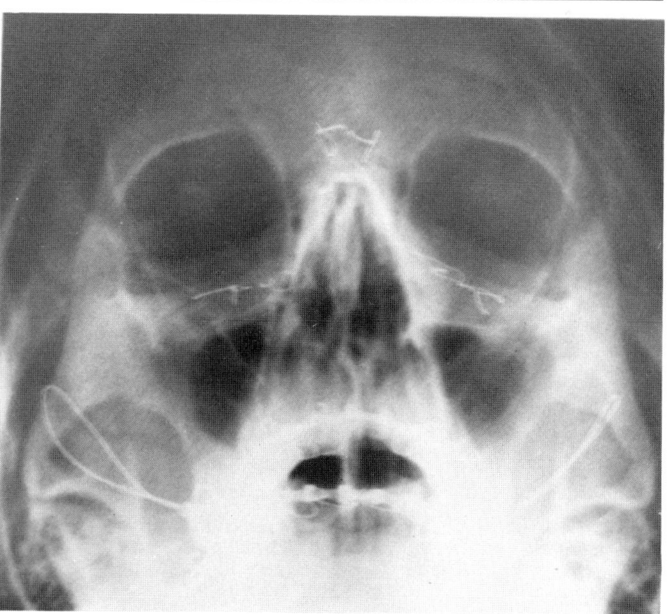

Figure 61C. Post reduction and fixation view.

orbital floor has been fractured and is displaced downward into the upper maxillary sinus. All of these features reflect that the force application was over the nasal arch, a little to the right of midline, and was directed obliquely downward and posteriorly in order to produce the resulting position of the main fragment.

After reduction and fixation of the orbital rim and nasal-frontal fractures, as well as arch bar application and interdental wiring, the resulting fragment position is almost anatomic as seen in Figure 61C. Slight caudal position of the left orbital floor remains. The surgeon chose to loop the right suspension wire over the zygomatic arch, while the left suspension wire was placed through the arch.

C. LeFort III Fracture

The true LeFort III fracture is very uncommon as an isolated injury. Fracture through this plane more commonly occurs as a unilateral part of the LeFort II-tripod injury, which will be described below under the LeFort variation portion. The LeFort III fracture may occur in association with severe skull injury, however.

The patient whose injury is demonstrated by Figure 62 had a severe head injury, which produced a temporoparietal fracture extending across the middle cranial fossa and sella. The blow also has resulted in a left mandible ramus fracture for which interdental wiring had already been done before the films were obtained. The lateral view in Figure 62A shows the temporo-parietal and transsella components of the injury. While partial reduction has occurred, the pterygomaxillary interruption is still evident. Figure 62B is a detail view of the temporal and sella changes in Figure 62A.

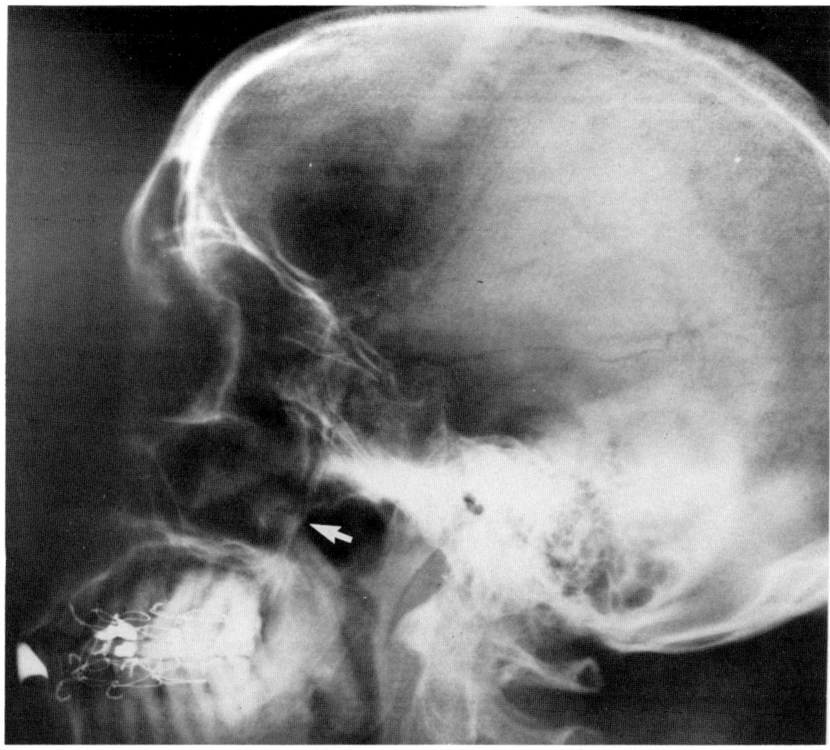

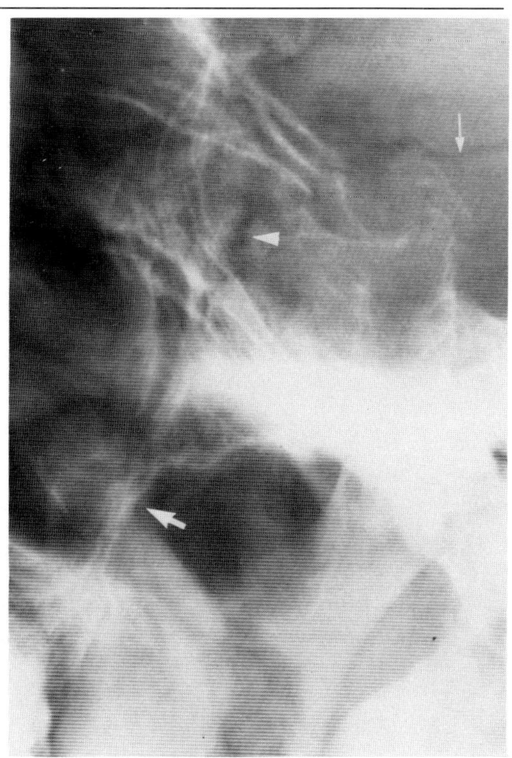

Figure 62A. LeFort III fracture. Lateral view with extensive temporoparietal and transsphenoidal fracture. Pterygoid process fracture at arrow.

Figure 62B. Detail view of Figure 62A.

Because of brain injury, only a tabletop anteroposterior Waters projection could be obtained. This view, Figure 62C, demonstrates a shift of the facial structures to the reader's left. An interrupted nasal arch is present, and both zygomatic arches are fractured just in front of the glenoid fossae. The inferior orbital rims and lateral maxillary walls are intact.

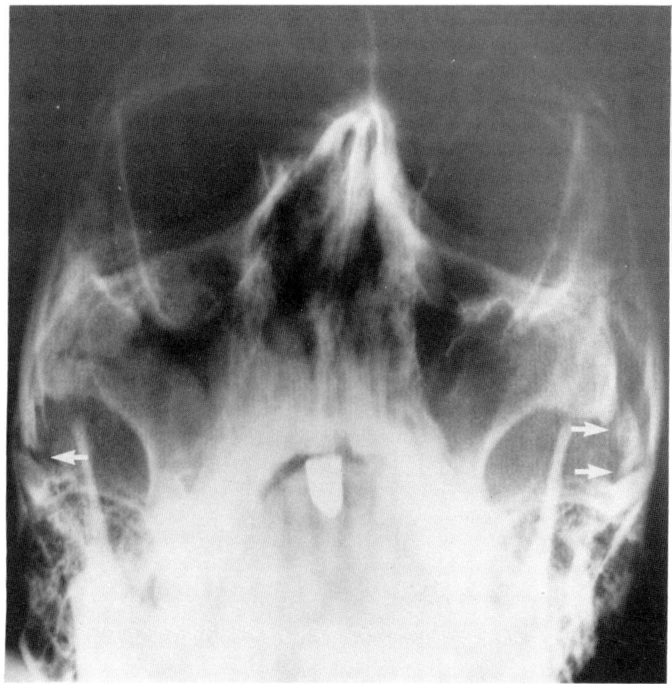

Figure 62C. Tabletop anteroposterior Waters view shows interrupted nasal arch and zygomatic arch fractures at arrows.

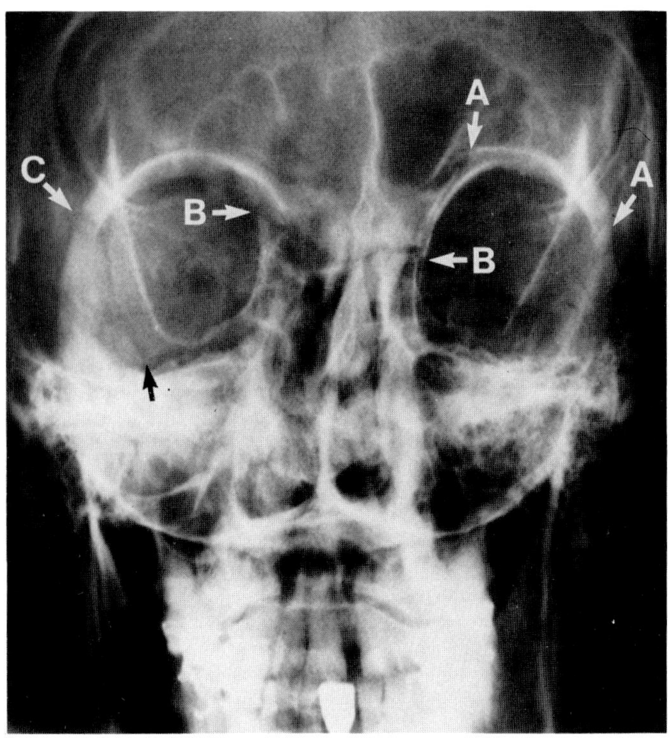

Figure 62D. Tabletop anteroposterior Caldwell view. Upper orbital rim fragment at A. Nasal-ethmoidal fracture at B. Suture separation and lateral orbital wall fracture at C.

A tabletop anteroposterior view in the Caldwell position is illustrated by Figure 62D. In this, a large left upper orbital rim fragment is present and is slightly rotated clockwise. The nasal-ethmoidal fracture is evident centrally. On the right, a zygomaticofrontal suture separation is present along with a perpendicular fracture through the lateral orbital wall. Shift of the upper facial fragment to the reader's left is again evident. Thus, the entire facial superstructure has been detached from its cranial attachments and has been displaced in position.

D. Tomography of LeFort Injuries

We employ tomography for the study of details of LeFort injury patterns. Figure 63A is a tomogram that shows a longitudinal hard palate fracture and right frontal fracture complicating a LeFort II injury pattern. Comminution of the left inferior orbital rim and lateral maxillary wall are also present.

If the presence or location of the pterygoid process fracture is not evident on plain films, tomography may be helpful. The patient illustrated in Figure 63B had bilateral pterygoid process fractures associated with a LeFort II injury.

The injury shown in Figure 63C was thought to represent a LeFort II injury on plain films. The tomographic study demonstrates that the fracture pattern is actually a LeFort I with a large left frontal process of maxilla fragment. The right nasal and orbital borders are intact on the tomographic study.

Tomography may also help illustrate orbital apex and optic canal injuries as we have seen in earlier sections of this book.

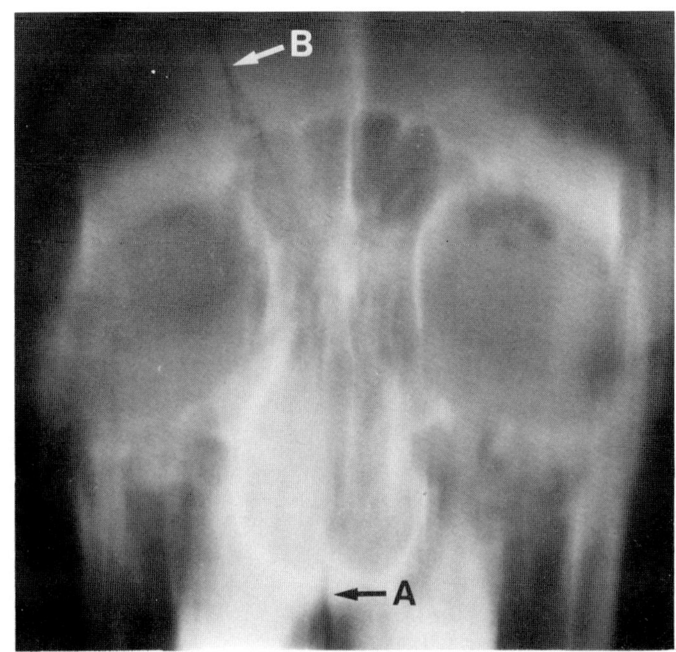

Figure 63A. Tomography as an adjunct means of evaluating LeFort injuries. Anteroposterior tomogram of a hard palate fracture at A and a right frontal fracture at B complicating a LeFort II injury.

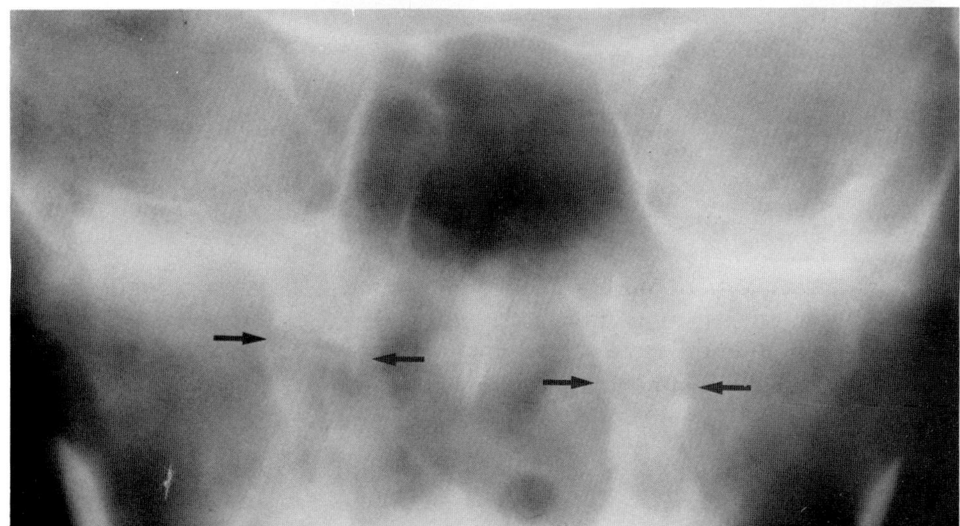

Figure 63B. Tomogram showing pterygoid process fractures (arrows) that were not evident on plain views.

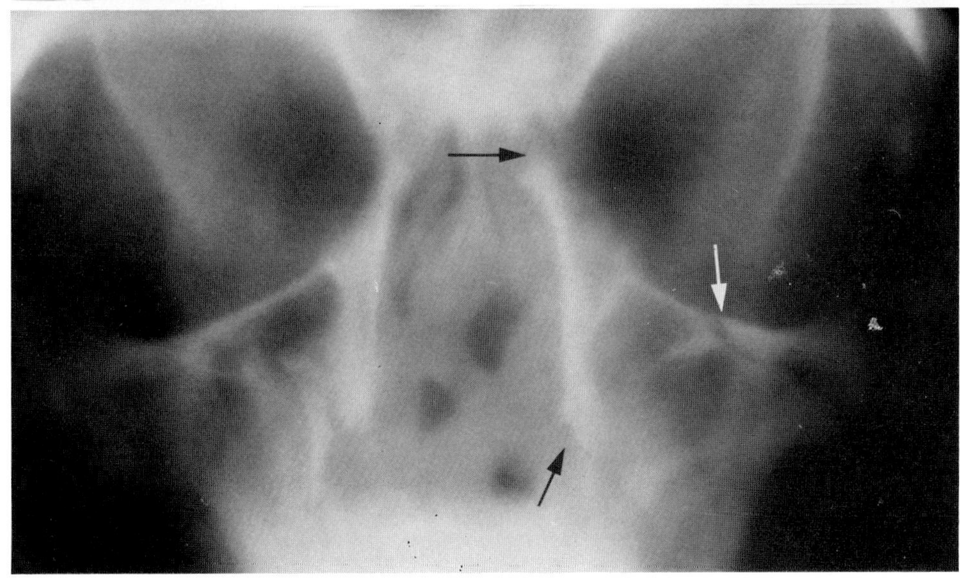

Figure 63C. LeFort I fracture with a large left frontal process fragment resembling a LeFort II fracture on plain films.

2. SPECIAL CONSIDERATIONS ABOUT LeFORT III FRACTURE COMPLEX

A. LeFort Fracture Variations

We have illustrated in Figure 63C how the large fragment LeFort injuries need not be symmetrical. This asymmetry is the principle variation in LeFort injury forms and may assume any right-sided and left-sided combination. These variations result from differences in the size and shape and in the direction and velocity of the injuring surface that comes into contact with the face. Perhaps one of the most frequent variations is the fracture in which a LeFort II fragment and a tripod fragment are produced by the same injury. This fracture form must be unique to those produced by a large amount of force, in that severe comminution is present at the contact location. These usually occur as a result of motor vehicle accidents and must therefore be the result of force application greater than that which LeFort could produce in the laboratory, for he did not describe this combination of injury among his induced fractures.

The Waters view in Figure 64A shows marked comminution in the nasal-ethmoidal area and along the left lateral maxillary border. On the right, the inferior orbital rim and lateral maxillary wall are separated in the LeFort II plane. This produces the central pyramidal fragment. In addition, a left tripod fragment results from separation of the zygomaticofrontal suture and lateral orbital wall, and the zygomatic arch is fractured near the glenoid fossa. The tripod fragment is displaced toward the patients' left side, while the LeFort fragment is displaced to the right.

Thus, in the LeFort II-tripod designation, we wish to call the attention of the surgeon to the two principal fragments that require stabilization.

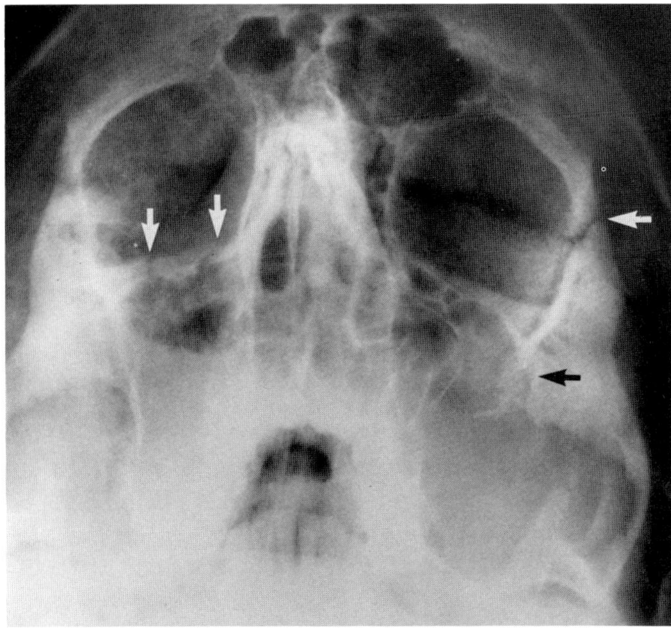

Figure 64A. A LeFort II-tripod fracture. Waters view with comminuted nasal arch and left maxillary border. Propagation fracture in the LeFort II plane on the right at vertical arrows. Left tripod fracture at horizontal arrows.

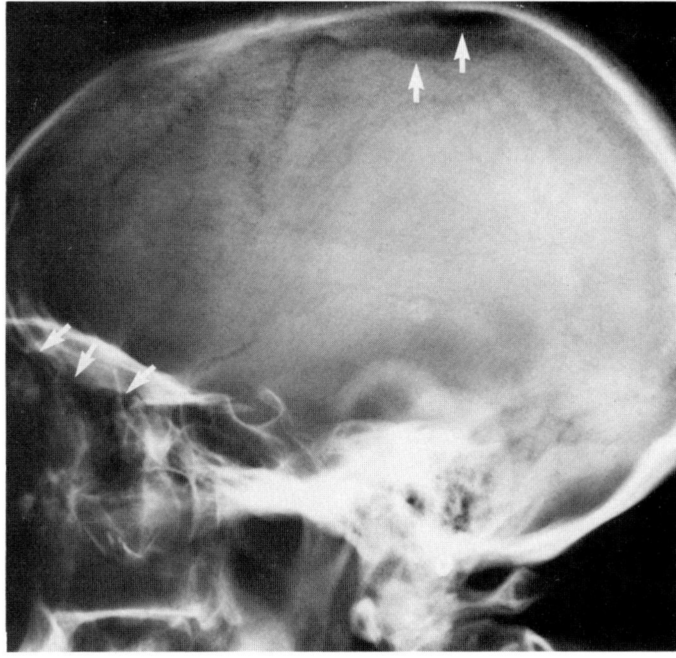

Figure 64B. Lateral view with pterygoid process and zygomatic recess fractures. Upper arrows on intracranial air-fluid levels. Lower arrows along ethmoidal roof (fovea) defect.

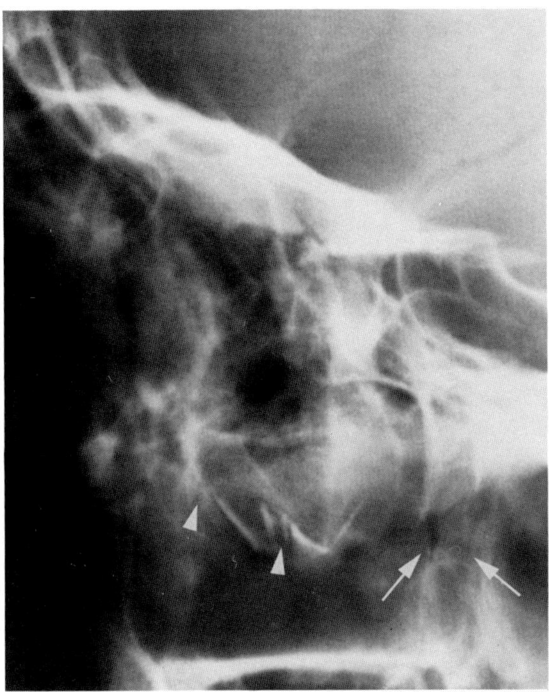

Figure 64C. Detail view of B.

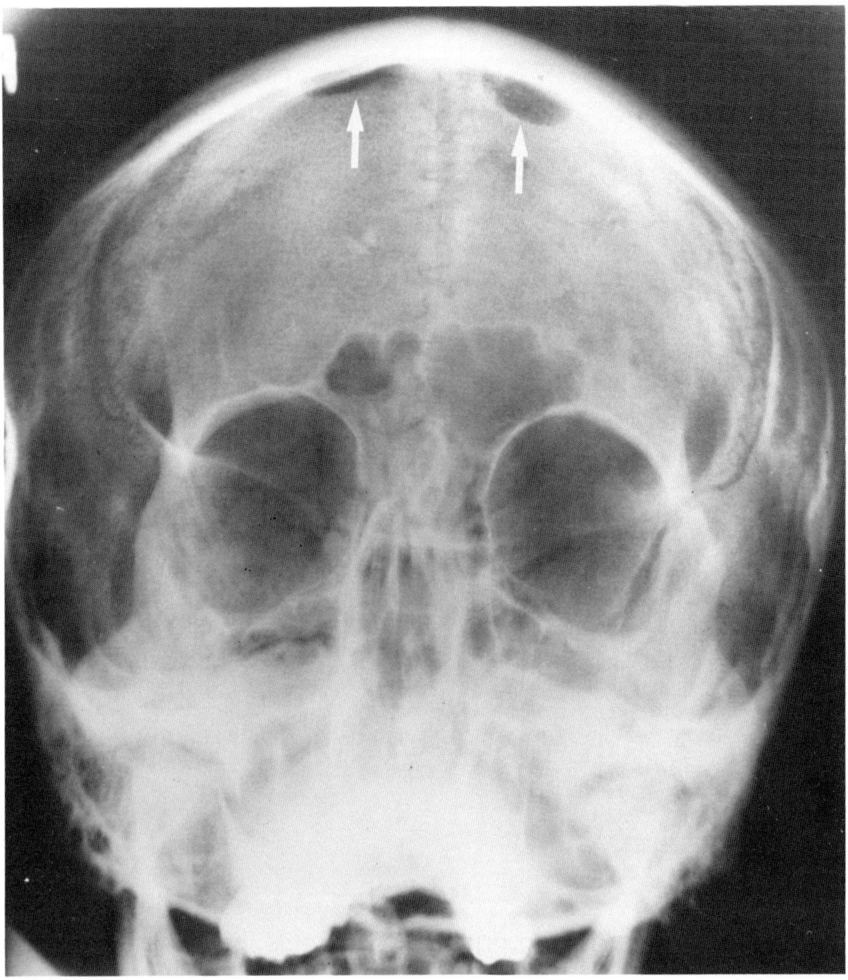

Figure 64D. Caldwell view with nasal arch comminution. Left lateral orbital wall fracture and intracranial air at arrows.

A second aspect of this fracture is the severe frontal or ethmoidal roof injury that frequently accompanies the LeFort II-tripod injury. In the lateral view, Figures 64B and C illustrate the posterior maxillary and pterygoid process fractures, as well as fractures of the zygomatic recess margins. Air-fluid levels can be seen in the high parasagittal region of the parietal area. This finding implies dural laceration with air escaping from a sinus cavity. If one carefully evaluates the lateral view, one finds no evidence of the ethmoidal roof. This reflects severe injury to the central portion of the anterior cranial fossa. A Caldwell view of this patient, Figure 64D, gives supplementary information regarding the nasal arch comminution, shows the left lateral orbital wall fracture, and confirms the intercranial location of the air.

CT is helpful in evaluating the presence of a LeFort II-tripod injury. Figure 65A is an axial CT through the midmaxilla. The right anterior and posterolateral maxillary borders have a fracture through the LeFort II plane. The right zygomatic arch was intact on serial views (not illustrated). A more comminuted LeFort II fracture is present in the left maxilla, and the zygomatic arch is bowed outward with fractures in the middle and preglenoid portions.

A higher view through the midorbit, Figure 65B, shows comminution and flattening of the nasal arch and maxillary frontal processes, as well as the left lateral orbit wall portion of the tripod fracture.

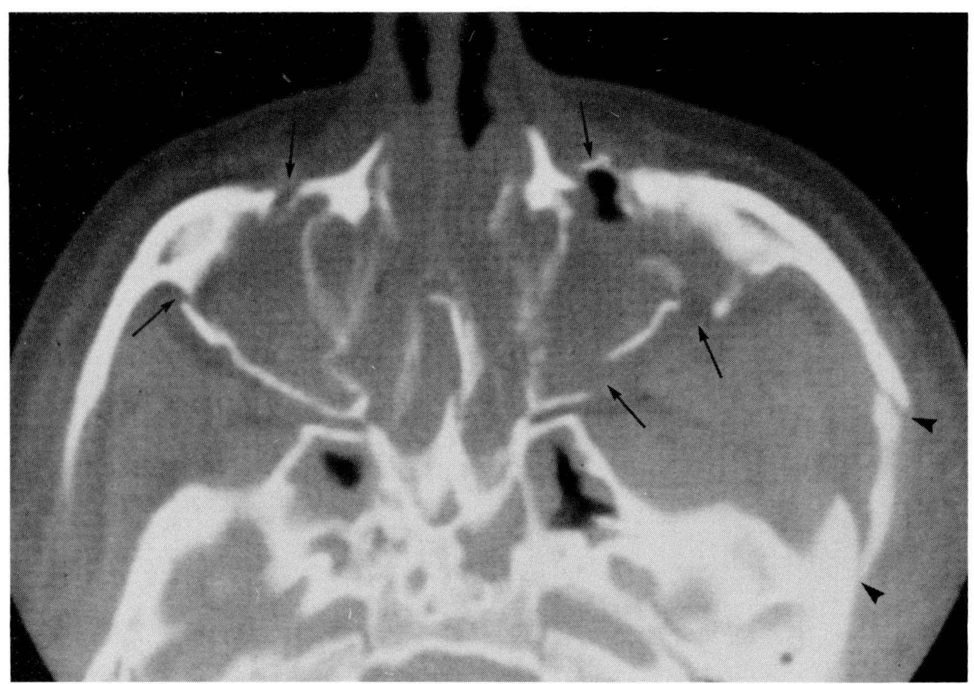

Figure 65A. CT of LeFort II-tripod fracture. Midmaxillary axial CT with maxillary wall LeFort II fractures bilaterally (arrows) and zygomatic arch fractures on the left (arrowheads).

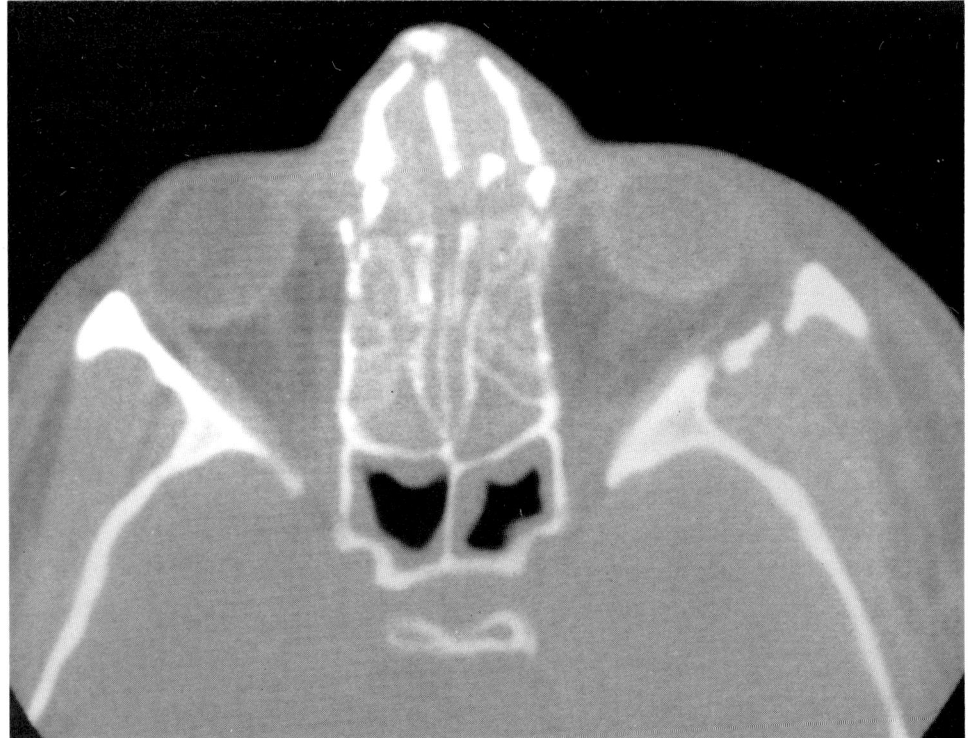

Figure 65B. Midorbit axial CT with nasal arch and frontal process fractures centrally (LeFort II) and left lateral orbit wall fractures (tripod).

B. LeFort II-Tripod and LeFort III Fracture Complex

If the contact location of a complex injury is above the nasal arch area, propagation of force may be along the LeFort III plane as seen in Figure 66. Force was applied over the left frontal, left zygomatic, and left mandibular area as seen in Figure 66A. This view also reveals a right-sided fracture in the LeFort III plane of weakness. An Erich arch bar with interdental wiring spans an oblique horizontal ramus mandible fracture that is not visible on this view. Resulting, therefore, is a large facial fragment that would be designated as a LeFort III-right and LeFort II-left plus a left tripod fragment as well. The proximal portion of the left zygomatic arch has also been sheared off through the glenoid fossa.

The right inferior orbital rim is intact in both the Waters view and the Caldwell view illustrated by Figure 66B. The large transfrontal fracture is also better seen in this view, as is the bilateral zygomaticofrontal suture separation.

A view of this patient after reduction and fixation is shown in Figure 66C. Wire sutures maintain the left orbital rim fracture. Zygomaticofrontal suture fixation has been achieved and incorporated with suspension wires, which are attached to surface buttons for easier removal after the suspension wires are no longer needed. An external T-shaped splint protects the frontal fracture.

While this fracture is clearly along the LeFort III plane of weakness on both sides, it would be insufficient to designate the fracture as such, for this would fail to call attention to the left inferior orbital rim and lateral maxillary wall fractures. Hence, the use of the more comprehensive term LeFort II-tripod for the injury on this side.

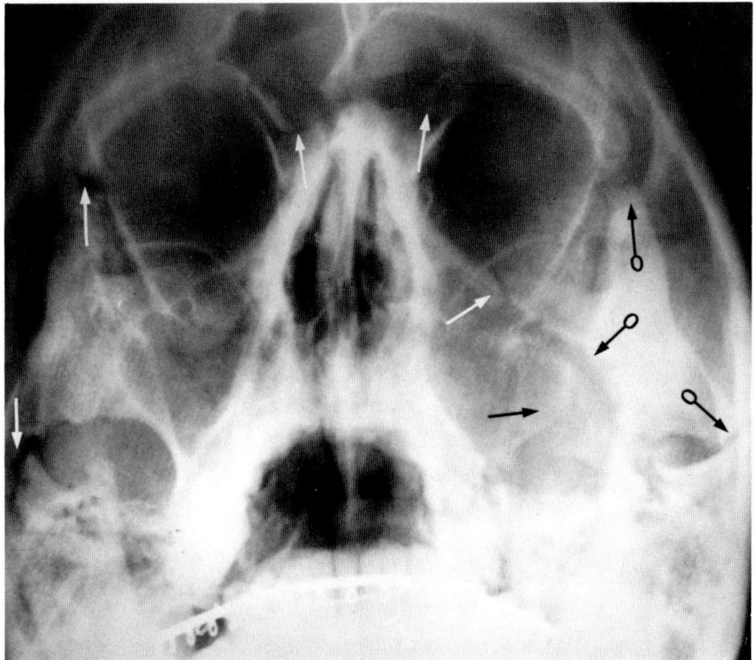

Figure 66A. Complex fracture consisting of a left LeFort II-tripod and right LeFort III interruption. Waters view showing a large fragment resulting from a right LeFort III fracture and a left LeFort II fracture. A left tripod fragment is also present. An Erich arch bar spans the mandibular teeth.

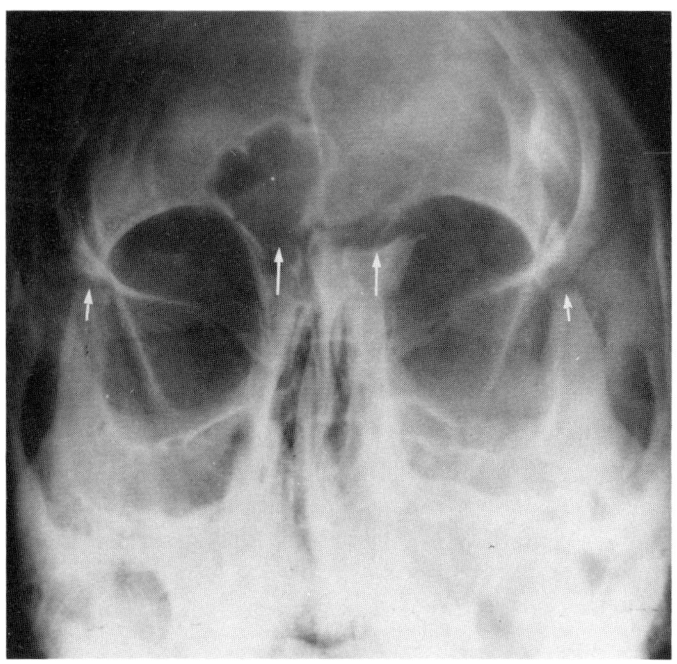

Figure 66B. The Caldwell view better defines the transfrontal and zygomaticofrontal suture separation.

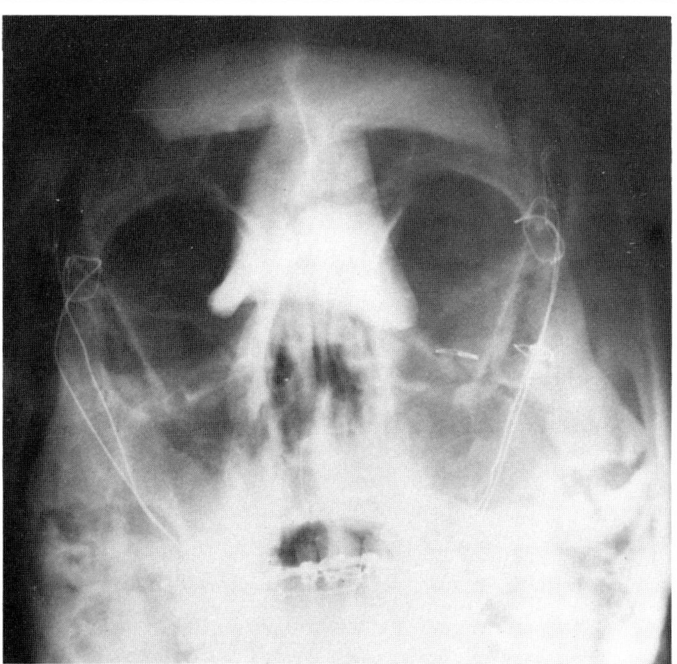

Figure 66C. Post reduction and fixation. Waters view.

C. Smash Fracture

The categorical term smash fracture is used by us to imply injury from application of great force producing rather complete comminution of all the facial structures. This term is usually modified to describe the portion of the face primarily involved. We use the terms *nasal-ethmoidal smash, frontal smash,* or *central facial smash* to describe the three major forms of this injury.

A secondary implication of this term is the likely association of injury to the underlying parts of the skull. Thus, in the case of the nasal-smash injury, one would expect ocular, orbital apex, and ethmoidal roof injury. Similarly, the frontal-smash injury implies an interruption of the frontal sinus walls and strongly suggests underlying dural and brain injury. In these fractures and in the central facial smash, the middle cranial fossa is injured, along with the sphenoidal sinus walls. Rarely, the accompanying basal skull fracture will extend into the temporal bone and produce facial, auditory, or vestibular nerve injury.

Those patients with a smash injury usually have not only skull fractures but also axial or peripheral skeletal injury as well. Because of the patient's unstable general condition or skeletal injury, it is usually impossible to obtain other than tabletop facial bone x-ray examination. Tomography may be a very helpful supplemental examination, and CT becomes especially useful for facial analysis and brain evaluation.

Figure 67A is the Waters view of a patient with a nasal-ethmoidal smash injury. In this, the nasal pyramid borders are hardly recognizable, and fractures through each of the vertical and horizontal facial buttresses are present. The Caldwell view of this patient in Figure 67B further illustrates the nasal-ethmoidal

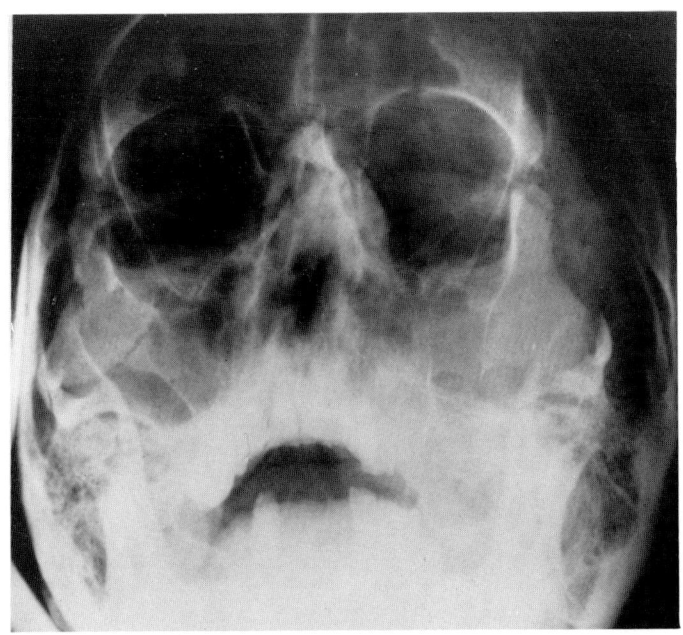

Figure 67A. Nasal-ethmoidal smash injury. Waters view.

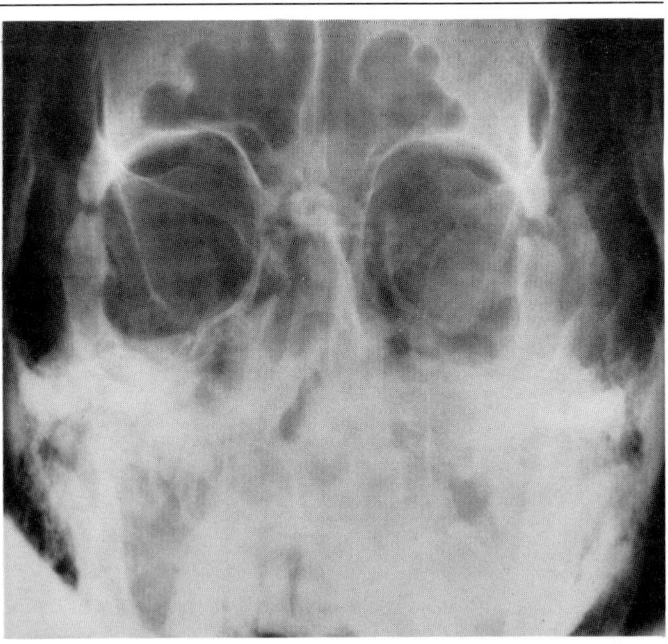

Figure 67B. Caldwell view.

comminution and reveals a small left frontal sinus air-fluid level. Bilateral zygomaticofrontal suture separation is present.

A frontal-smash injury is shown in Figure 68. The frontal sinus walls were comminuted and had been decompressed by the time a lateral view, Figure 68A, could be obtained. Ethmoidal roof interruption and an opaque sphenoidal sinus are also evident in this view.

Figure 68B is a tabletop anteroposterior view of the same patient. All of the facial buttresses have been interrupted. A posteroanterior view after reduc-

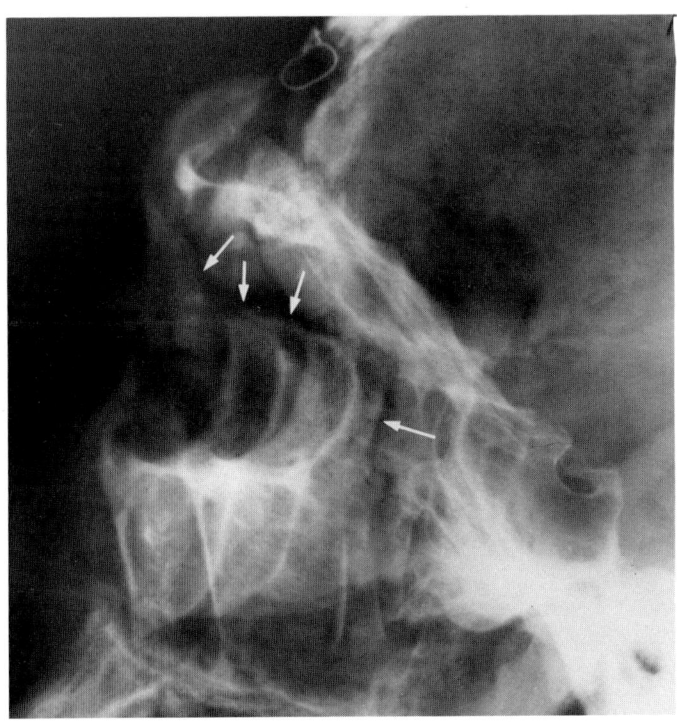

Figure 68A. Frontal-smash injury. Lateral view.

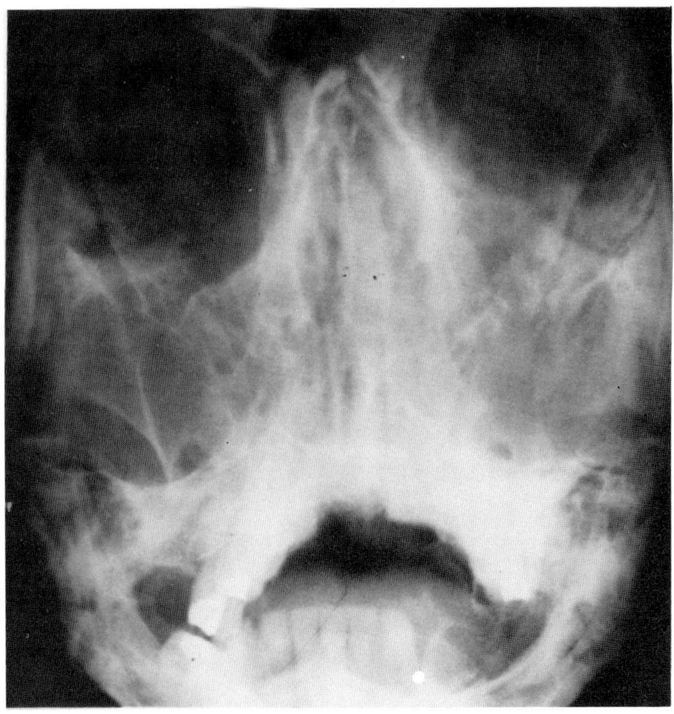

Figure 68B. Tabletop anteroposterior Waters view.

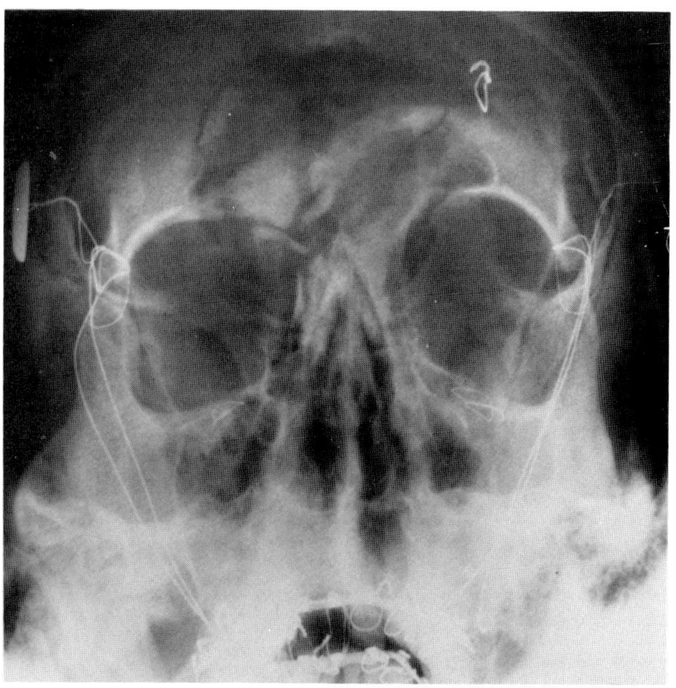

Figure 68C. Postoperative. Waters view.

tion and fixation is illustrated in Figure 68C. Obvious distortion of the frontal sinus, nasal arch, and left orbit persist, and these patients often need extensive cosmetic surgical repair following such a devastating injury.

Only emergency survey anteroposterior and lateral views were available to illustrate the plain film findings of the central facial smash injury in Figure 69A. This view shows extensive frontal and right orbital comminution. The lateral facial view in Figure 69B demonstrates complete frontal, orbital roof, and ethmoidal roof interruption, as well as comminution of all facial bones. An anteroposterior tomogram after frontal decompression and interdental wiring is shown in Figure 69C. Comminution of the entire facial skeleton is present.

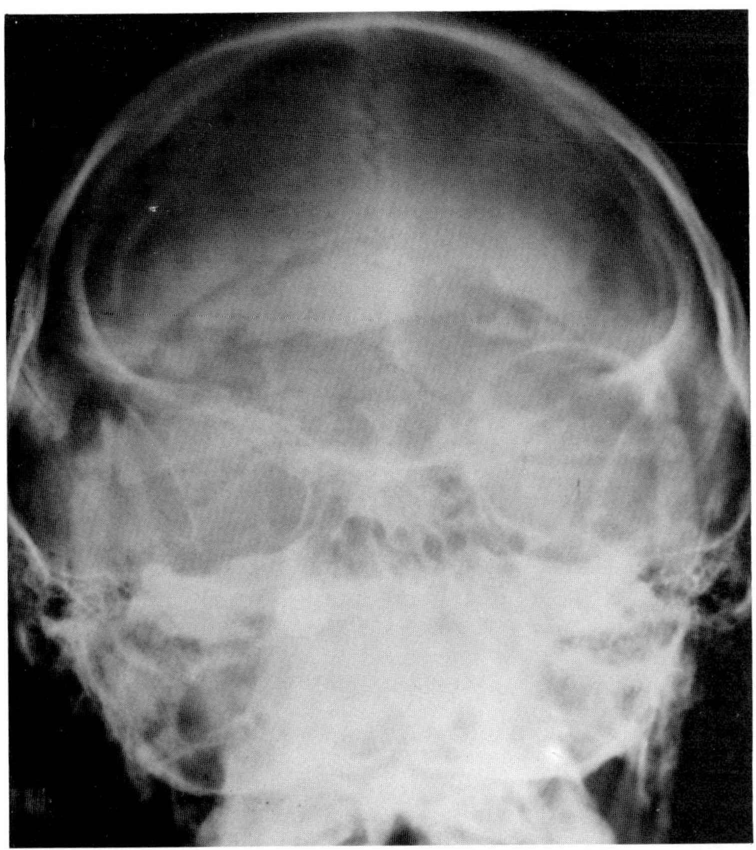

Figure 69A. Central facial smash injury. Survey tabletop anteroposterior view.

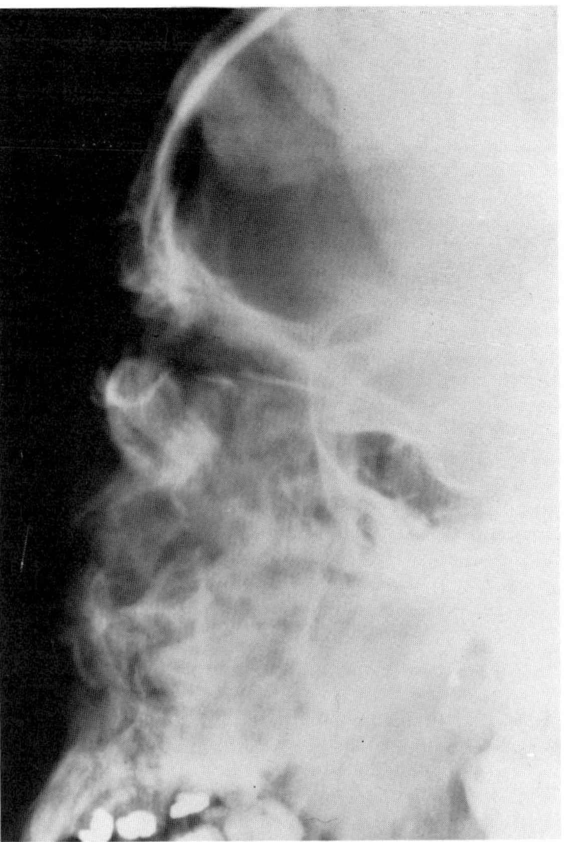

Figure 69B. Survey lateral facial view.

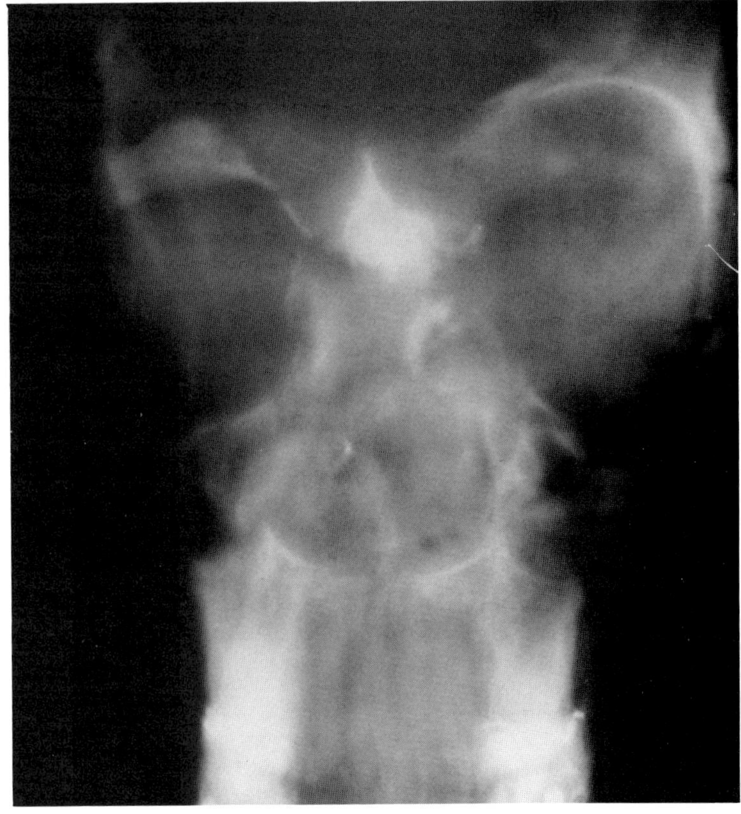

Figure 69C. Anterior facial tomogram.

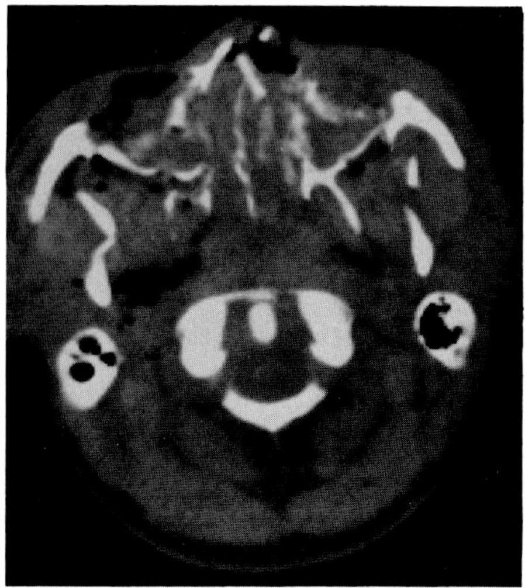 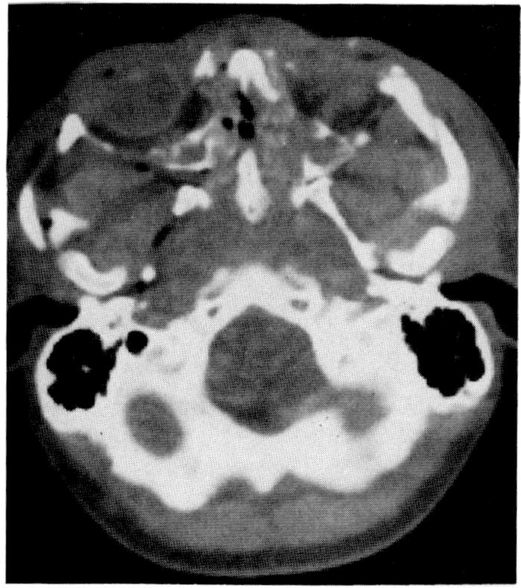 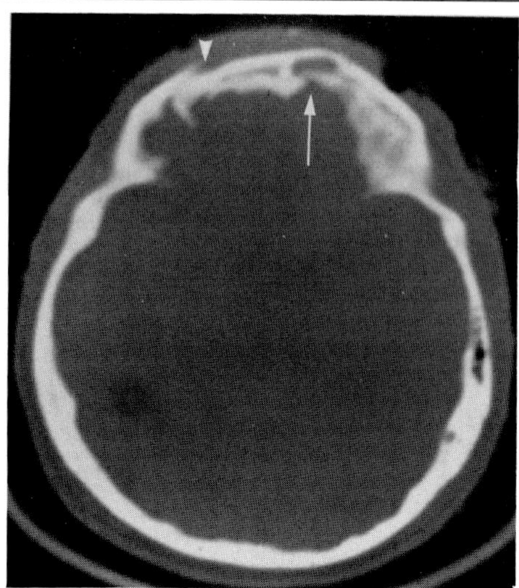

Figures 69D–F. Central facial smash injury. (D) Transmaxillary CT (bone window). (E) Transorbital CT (bone window). (F) Transfrontal CT (bone window).

Figure 69D is an axial CT through the midmaxillary plane showing extensive comminution of the facial bones with posterior compressive displacement. The sinuses are opaque, and air is present in the subcutaneous, retromaxillary, and right parapharyngeal areas. The nasopharynx is obscured by blood.

A transorbital CT in Figure 69E illustrates posterior displacement of the nasal arch and total facial bone disruption. Rupture of the left eye is present.

Figure 69F is an axial CT through the frontal sinus. A depressed fracture is present just lateral to the right sinus border. An oblique fracture extends through the left frontal sinus, and a deep cutaneous laceration is present just lateral to the left frontal sinus.

6

Supplementary Studies to Evaluate Intracranial Injury Accompanying Facial Trauma

The relationship of facial injury and intracranial injury has not been studied in a correlative fashion so that prevalance statistics are not available. We do know that closed cranial trauma may occur without overt injury to the scalp or calvaria. Therefore, the clinician must depend on his neurologic evaluation of the patient along with a strong sense of suspicion in connection with injury about the head in order to detect intracranial complications and brain injury.

The presence of a specific skull base fracture on radiologic examination should strongly suggest an injury of the brain or meninges. Since the anterior and middle cranial fossae may be injured with the more severe facial fractures, it is appropriate to provide a few examples of the use of brain CT in evaluating such injuries.

The patient shown in Figure 70 had a severe orbital roof and frontal sinus injury following a car accident. Figure 70A shows the comminuted fracture of the anterior frontal sinus wall to be a depressed fracture. A prominent posterior sinus wall step-off is also present. Meningeal injury was suspected. Therefore, the CT examination was carried to the upper surface of the calvarium. Only the highest axial CT views showed intracranial air as seen in Figure 70B. The meningeal air implies infection may occur.

A similar, but less depressed frontal-orbital fracture was found in the examination illustrated by Figure 71. Accompanying the frontal sinus wall fracture is a more lateral fracture extending from the orbit roof into the frontal surface of the skull. Figure 71A is an axial CT using bone window setting that shows the fractures. A companion axial CT of the same section using a soft tissue window shows a supraorbital epidural hematoma along with compressive change of the anterior horns of the lateral ventricles. This is illustrated by Figure 71B.

A sphenoid wing fracture is illustrated in Figure 72. The fracture was produced by a blow from the lateral direction and involves both the outer surface of the greater wing and orbital apex as demonstrated in Figure 72A. Since the patient also had clinical signs of increased intracranial pressure, an unenhanced brain CT study was also performed. A large blood accumulation

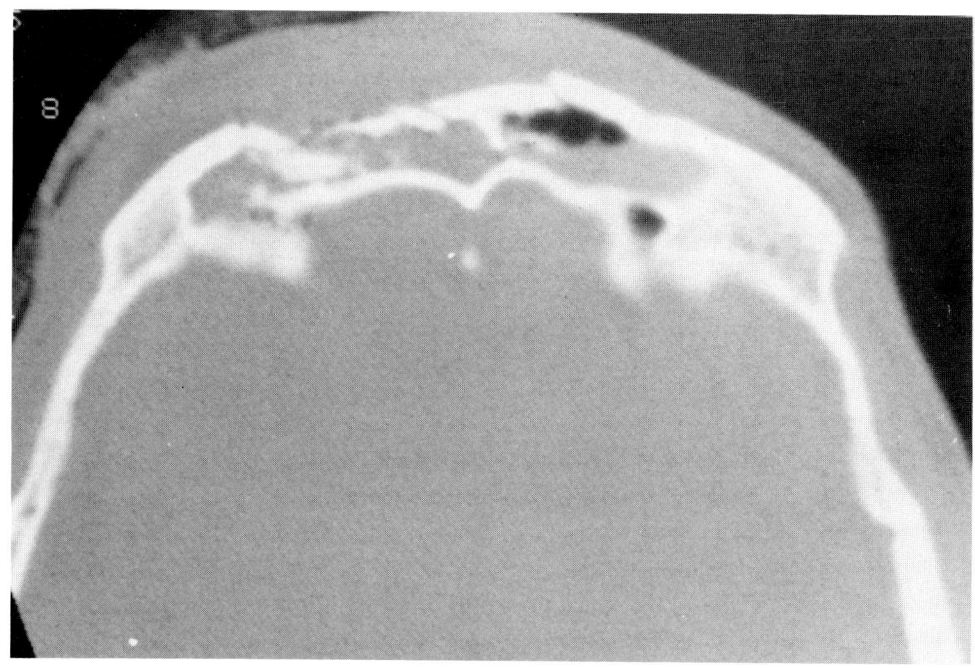

Figure 70A. Intracranial subarachnoid air associated with an orbital roof and depressed frontal sinus fracture. Low frontal axial CT demonstrates the frontal sinus anterior and posterior wall fractures.

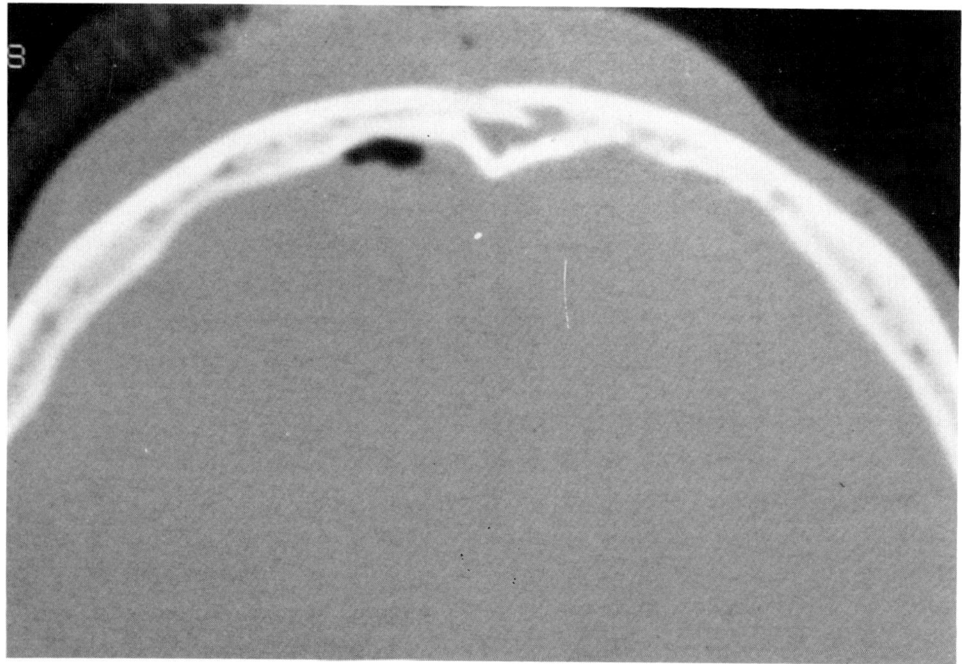

Figure 70B. A high axial frontal bone CT shows an intracranial air accumulation.

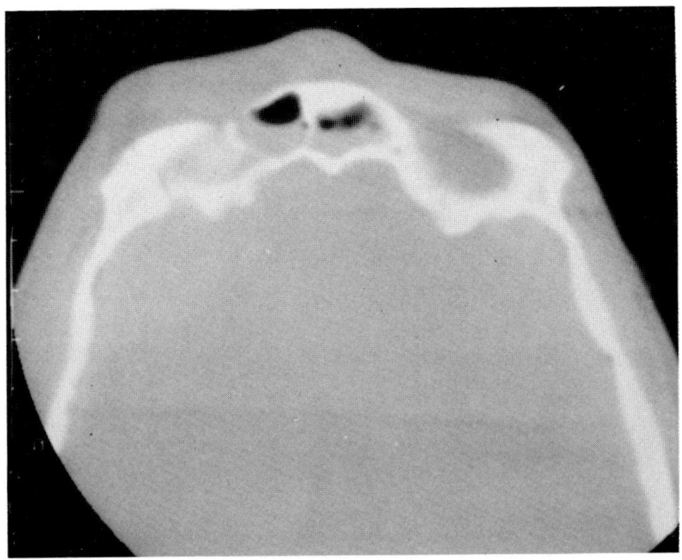

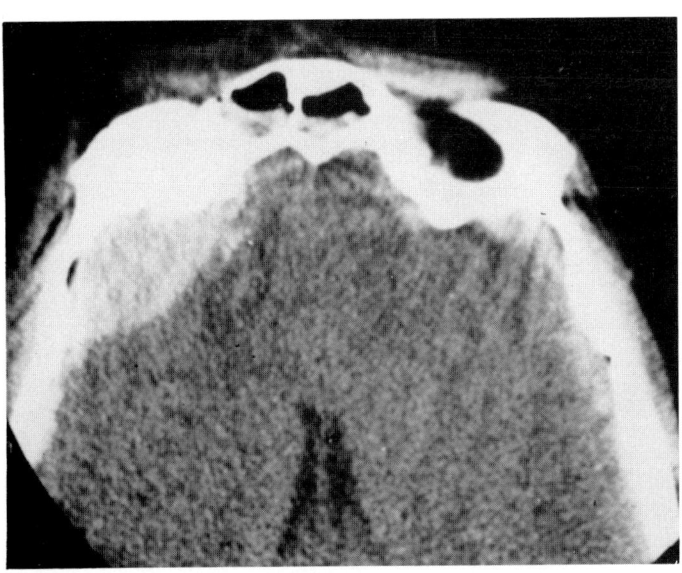

Figure 71A. Frontal sinus and frontal bone fracture complicated by an epidural hematoma. Bone window axial CT shows the right-side sinus and frontal bone fractures.

Figure 71B. Soft tissue window axial CT of the same segment shows the epidural blood collection just above orbit roof.

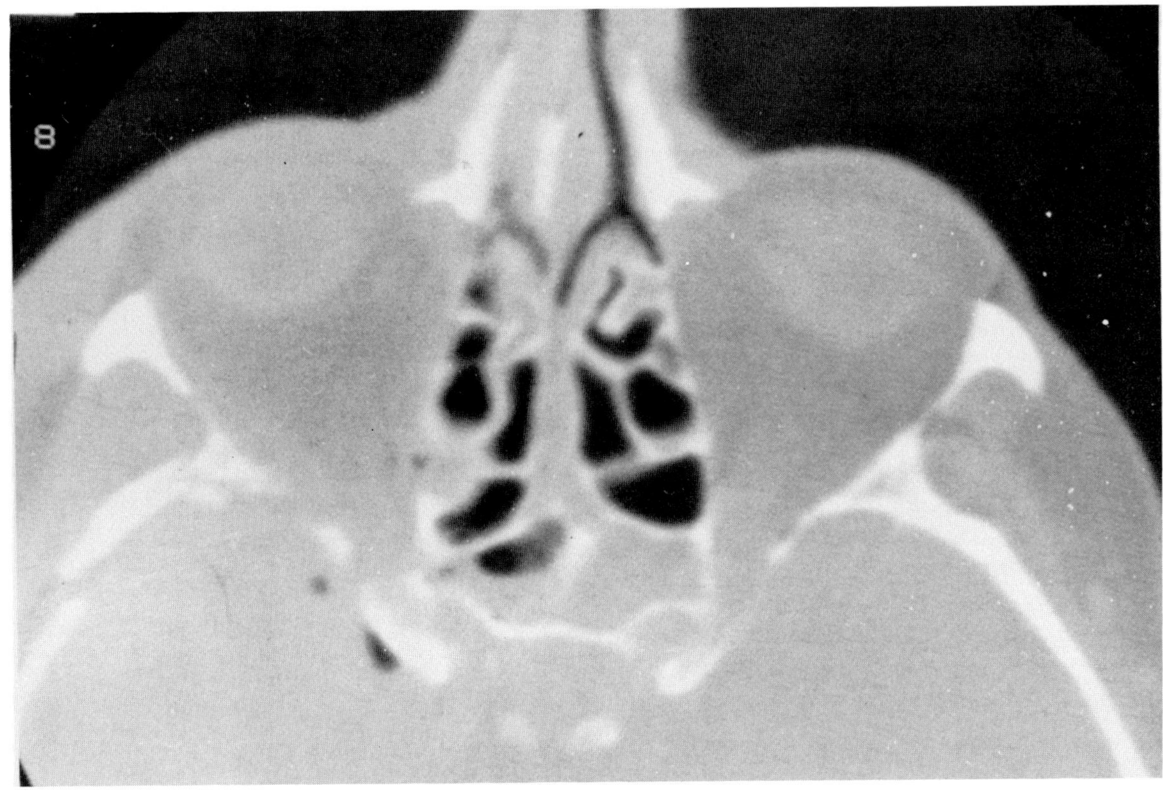

Figure 72A. Right sphenoid wing and orbit fractures complicated by an intracranial hemorrhage. A midorbit axial CT shows the right orbit apex and lateral greater wing fractures.

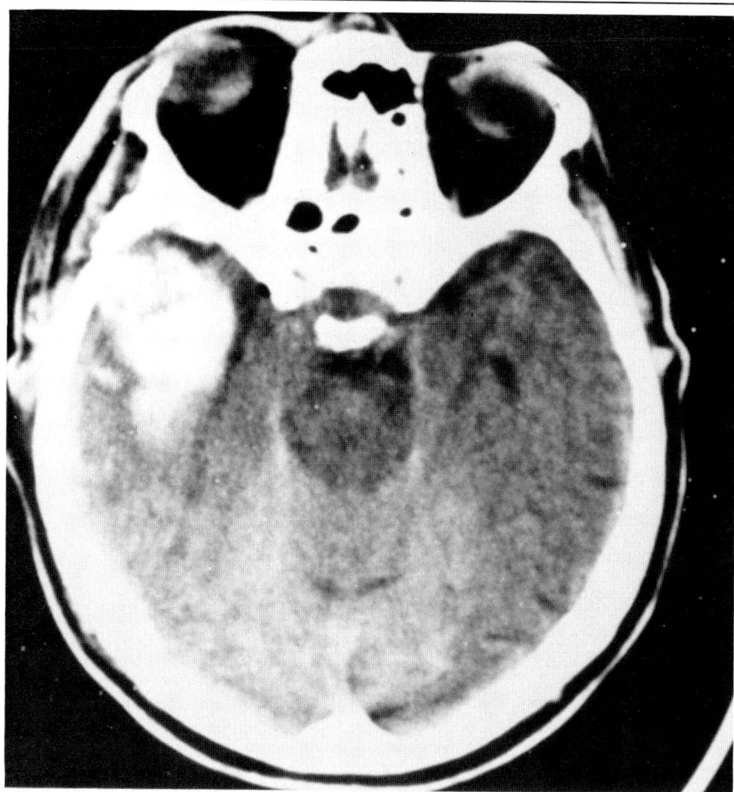

Figure 72B. An unenhanced brain CT at a slightly higher level than in Figure 72A shows a large temporal lobe and sylvian sulcus hematoma.

was present in the underlying temporal lobe and sylvian sulcus as seen in Figure 72B.

Magnetic resonance (MR) examination will probably play an increasing role in studying specific intracranial problems associated with facial injury. The patient in Figure 73 had an undisplaced left tripod fracture with an accompanying linear fracture of the orbit roof on plain films. Marked reduction in visual acuity was present. A midorbit axial CT represented by Figure 73A shows periorbital preseptal swelling, an opaque left ethmoid sinus, and soft tissue "fullness" in the orbit apex. This suggested, but did not define, optic nerve compression.

Examination of the orbit and brain using magnetic resonance (TR-1000 MS and TE-40 MS) shows a hematoma compressing the orbital muscle conus at the apex on the side of the ethmoid injury as illustrated in Figure 73B. We believe magnetic resonance studies will result in more precise information about complications in facial injury. Surface coil technology will allow even better anatomic representation than that presented in this case.

One final case demonstrates the advantage of magnetic resonance over CT in evaluating brain injury. The patient illustrated by Figure 74 had a left LeFort II-tripod fracture as well as a depressed left temporal fossa lateral wall fracture. A transorbital axial CT view is shown in Figure 74A, where ethmoid and sphenoid sinus opacity and middle cranial fossa air accompany the fracture through the left middle fossa wall. Conventional unenhanced brain CT examination revealed punctate hemorrhagic areas consistent with contusion

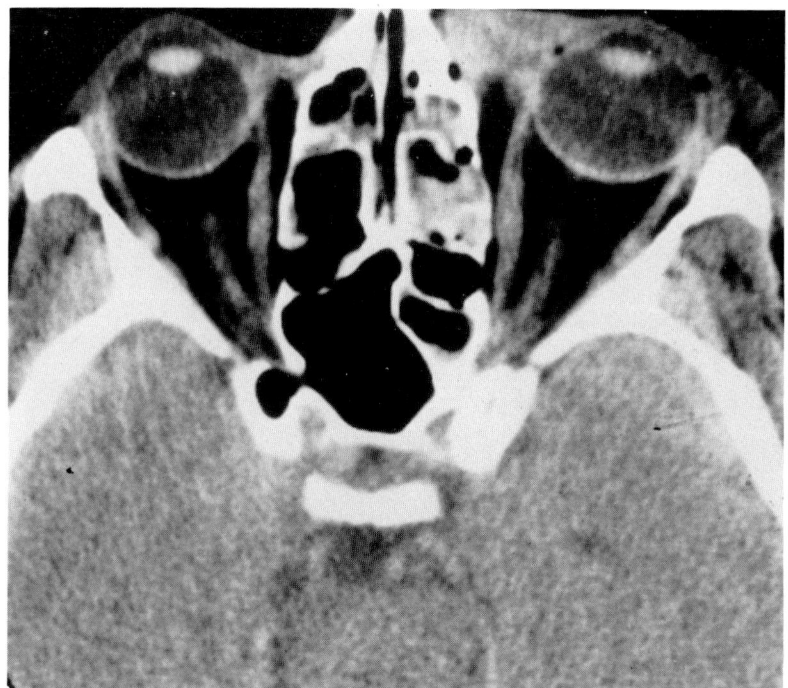

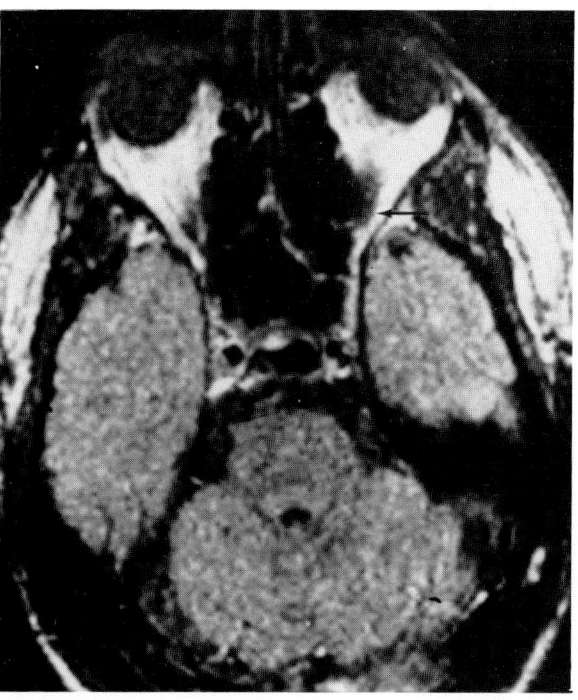

Figure 73A. Orbit apex hematoma producing optic nerve compression. Midorbit axial CT with left preseptal swelling, ethmoid sinus opacity, and questionable orbit apex hematoma.

Figure 73B. T$_1$-weighted magnetic resonance study with compressive change in the orbit apex (arrow).

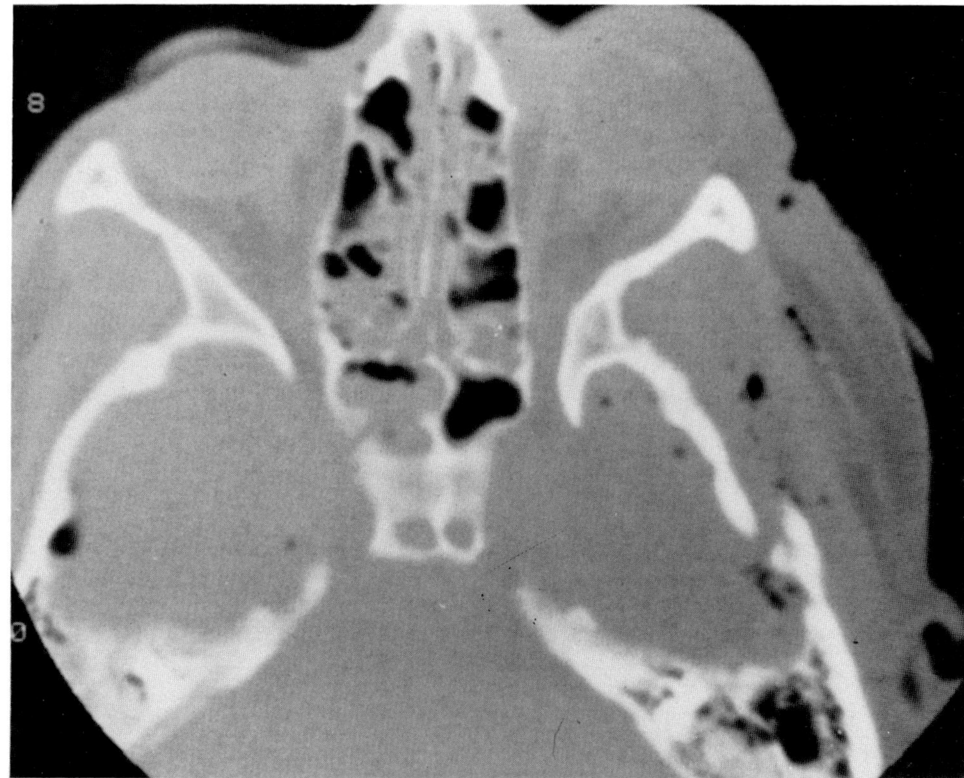

Figure 74A. LeFort II-left tripod and left lateral middle fossa fracture. Midorbit axial CT with ethmoid and sphenoid sinus opacity, middle fossa air, and left lateral wall temporal fossa fracture.

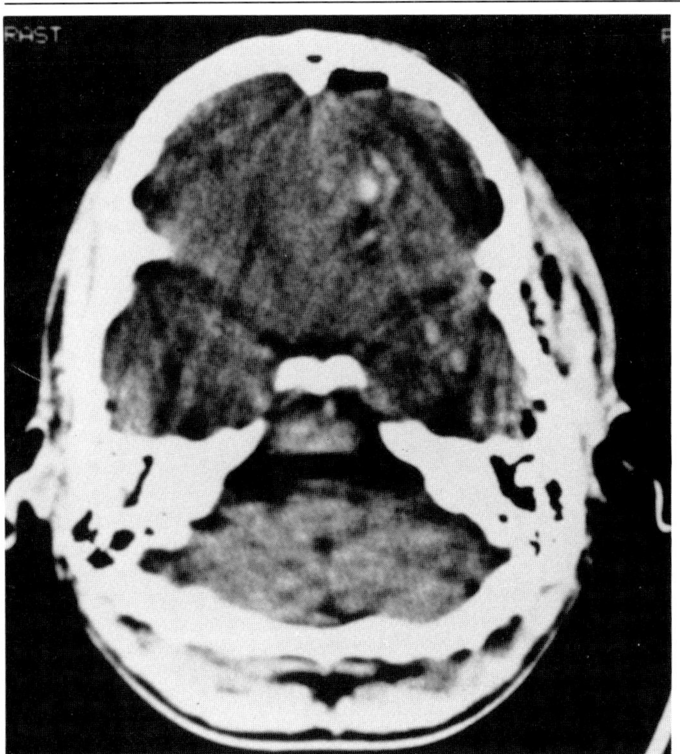

Figure 74B. Unenhanced axial brain CT with focal hemorrhages in the frontal and temporal lobes suggesting contusion.

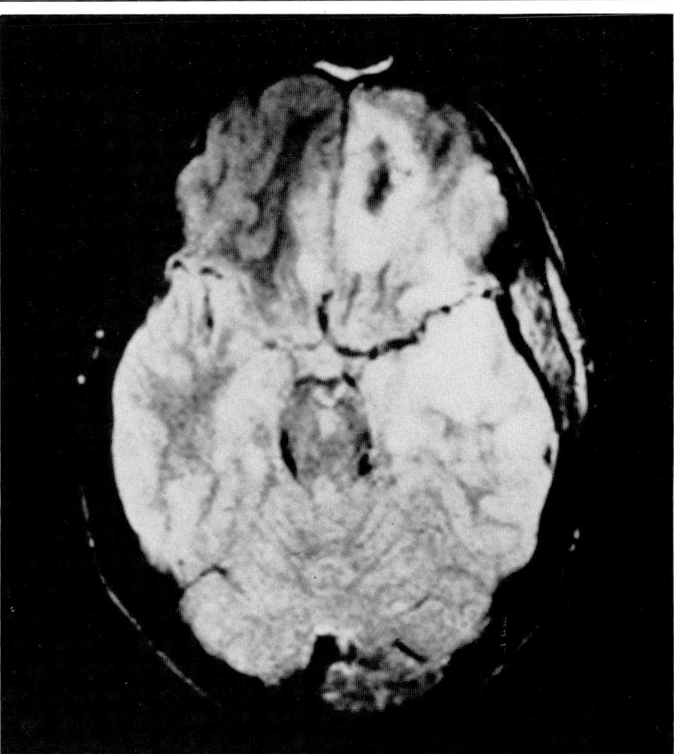

Figure 74C. T_2-weighted MR study (TR-2300 ms and TE-80 ms) showing much more brain injury than indicated by CT.

in the left frontal and temporal lobes as illustrated in Figure 74B. The CT study did not match the degree of coma, so magnetic resonance studies were performed, A T_2-weighted scan at the level of circle of Willis, Figure 74C, gives a better representation of the left frontal lobe and temporal lobe hemorrhage and edema. A small pontine hemorrhage is also present centrally.

These cases illustrate a preliminary impression of the application of MR in the study of soft tissue injury. As our collective national experience in MR broadens, we feel that wider use of this modality in studying brain injury will occur.

Suggested Readings

1. Dolan KD Fracturas maxilofaciales. Revista Mexicana de Radiol 1971; 25:89−103.
2. Dolan KD, Jacoby CG. Facial fractures. Semin Roentgenol 1978; 13:37−51.
3. Emery JM, VonNoorden GK, Schlernitzauer DA. Orbital floor fractures. Trans Am Acad Opth Oto 1971; 75:802−812.
4. Erkonen W, Dolan KD. Ocular Foreign Body Localization. Rad Clin North Am 1972; 10:101−104.
5. Gentry LR, Manor WF, Turski PA, Strother CM. High-resolution CT analysis of facial struts in trauma: 1. Normal anatomy. AJR 1983; 140:523−532.
6. Gentry LR, Manor WF, Turski PA, Strother CM. High-resolution CT analysis of facial struts in trauma: 2. Osseous and soft tissue complications. AJR 1983; 140:533−542.
7. Hammerschlag SB, Hughes S, O'Reilly GV, Weber AL. Another look at the blowout fractures of the orbit. AJNR 1982; 3:331−335.
8. McCoy FJ, Chandler RA, Magnan CG, Moore JR, Siemsen G. An analysis of facial fractures and their complications. Plastic Reconstructive Surg 1962; 29:381−391.
9. Nakamura T, Gross CW. Facial fractures. Arch Otolaryngol 1973; 97:288−290.
10. Rogers LF. *Radiology of Skeletal Trauma*. Churchill Livingstone, Inc. New York, NY 1982; 229−272.
11. Schultz RC, Oldham RJ. An overview of facial injuries. Surg Clin North Am 1977; 57:987−1010.
12. Tilson HB, McFee AS, Soudah HP. *Maxillo-Facial Works of René LeFort*. The University of Texas, Houston, TX, 1972.
13. Turvey TA. Midfacial fractures. J Oral Surg 1977; 35:887−891.

Index